SPRINGHOUSE **CLINICAL ROTATION GUIDES**™

Maternal-Newborn Nursing
Second Edition

Mary Dirr Kostenbauder, RN, CNM, MEd, MSN
Professor
Seminole Community College
Sanford, Florida

Springhouse Corporation
Springhouse, Pennsylvania

Staff For This Volume

Executive Director, Editorial
Stanley Loeb

Senior Publisher, Trade and Textbooks
Minnie B. Rose, RN, BSN, MEd

Art Director
John Hubbard

Editors
Diane Labus, David Moreau

Clinical Consultants
Patricia Kardish Fischer, RN, BSN;
Maryann Foley, RN, BSN

Copy Editors
Diane M. Armento, Debra Davis,
Pamela Wingrod

Designers
Stephanie Peters (associate art director), Amy Smith (senior designer), Janice Nawn

Typography
Diane Paluba (manager), Elizabeth Bergman, Joyce Rossi Biletz, Phyllis Marron, Robin Mayer, Valerie L. Rosenberger

Manufacturing
Deborah Meiris (director), Anna Brindisi, T.A. Landis

Editorial Assistants
Caroline Lemoine, Louise Quinn, Betsy K. Snyder

Printed in the United States of America. For information, write Springhouse Corporation, 1111 Bethlehem Pike, P.O. Box 908, Springhouse, PA 19477-0908. CRG4-020796

A member of the Reed Elsevier plc group

Library of Congress Cataloging-in-Publication Data
Kostenbauder, Mary Dirr.
    Maternal-newborn nursing / Mary Dirr Kostenbauder. — 2nd ed.
        p. cm. — (Clinical rotation guides)
    Includes bibliographical references and index.
    1. Maternity nursing — Handbooks, manuals, etc.   2. Infants (Newborn) — Diseases — Nursing — Handbooks, manuals, etc.   I. Title.
    II. Series: Springhouse clinical rotation guides.
    [DNLM: 1. Maternal-Child Nursing — handbooks.
    WY 39 K86m 1995]
RG951.K65   1995
610.73'678 — dc20
DNLM/DLC   94-32667
ISBN 0-87434-734-3   CIP

Table of Contents

Consultants, Acknowledgment, and Dedication

Series Consulting Editor
Mary Jane Evans, RN, BSN
Independent Consultant for Nursing Education
Winter Park, Florida

Clinical Consultant
Corey H. Evans, MD
Associate Director
Family Practice Residency
Florida Hospital
Orlando

Acknowledgment
Thanks to Ruth Wallace, RNC, and Maureen Daniels, ARNP, for their consultation during the preparation of this second edition.

Dedication
To the memory of my father, Albert Dirr, who taught me to have faith in God, to spend time with my children, and to love animals. These things have given meaning and balance to my life.

Preface

Maternal-Newborn Nursing, Second Edition will assist the student in planning and implementing care of the childbearing family in the clinical setting. Developed as a supplementary aid, it in no way substitutes for an in-depth study of maternal-newborn care; rather, it provides quick access to information useful to nursing students on maternal-newborn clinical rotations.

Within this book, the student will find clinical instruction on:
• performing a nursing assessment of the maternity patient and her newborn
• understanding the essential concepts behind frequently used obstetric terminology
• identifying nursing diagnoses and interventions associated with the normal course of pregnancy and with the more common complications encountered during the childbearing process
• assisting with and performing procedures and diagnostic tests specific to maternal-newborn care.

1 Assessing the Normal Childbearing Family

As part of your clinical rotation, you will be expected to partici-pate in caring for the maternity patient and her newborn infant. This section offers specific information on how to assess and care for both of them — from the initial assessment to the post-delivery period.

☐ Initial prenatal assessment

During the first prenatal visit, you'll need to take a detailed, com-prehensive patient history, assess the patient's emotional and edu-cational level, and anticipate her needs during the childbearing cycle. Although you'll be gathering much data during this ses-sion, keep in mind that the assessment will continue throughout the prenatal period. Also during this initial visit, the patient will undergo a physical examination.

Taking the nursing history
When taking the history, be sure to record all pertinent informa-tion carefully, as this serves as the basis on which the patient's prenatal care is planned. Depending on your clinical setting, you'll probably record the data on an assessment form.

General patient information
Carefully document the following information:

Patient's age
Patients at the extremes of the usual childbearing age-group (teenagers, those over age 35) are at increased risk for certain complications, including pregnancy-induced hypertension (PIH) and preterm labor. Any patient who will be age 35 at the time of delivery should be offered the option of genetic counseling be-cause of the increased risk of chromosomal anomalies.

Race and ethnic origin
Blacks and persons of Mediterranean ancestry should be screened for sickle cell trait or disease. Women of Greek, Italian, Chinese, Southeast Asian, African, and Mediterranean descent are at increased risk for thalassemia, an inherited disorder of hemoglobin synthesis. Jews should be screened for Tay-Sachs disease. Haitians, Africans, Asians, Inuits, and women from the Pacific Basin should be screened to deter-mine if they are a chronic carrier of hepatitis B.

Religion
Certain religious groups, such as Jehovah's Witnesses, adhere to

beliefs that may interfere with medical treatment. These patients should be questioned about receiving blood products.

Occupation

Various occupations (whether current or former) may place the patient or her infant at risk. The following workers may be exposed to chemicals or infectious agents:
- textile operators
- upholsterers
- sewers and stitchers
- doctors, nurses, aides, and orderlies
- dentists; dental hygienists, assistants, and technicians
- laboratory workers
- electronic assemblers
- hairdressers and cosmetologists
- launderers and dry cleaners
- photographic processors
- plastic fabricators
- agricultural workers
- transportation operators
- sign painters and letterers
- clerical personnel
- opticians and lens grinders
- printing operators.

Marital status, years married

Single women may be at increased risk for preterm labor because of socioeconomic factors and may need additional emotional support in dealing with the pregnancy and in responding to the demands of parenting. Couples who have been married for several years before the birth of their first child may also need additional emotional support in adapting their lifestyle to the demands of parenting.

Support systems available during pregnancy are important. Because of the high incidence of spouse abuse and its escalation during pregnancy, the nurse should be aware of possible signs of battering.

Education (highest grade completed)

Women with less than a high school education have shown an increased risk for preterm labor, probably as a result of socioeconomic factors. Knowing this will also help you in adapting educational activities to meet the needs of individual patients.

Age and health of the baby's father

Men over age 50 may be at increased risk for fathering children with chromosomal defects. Significant information regarding the father's health includes his present general state of health and his history of drug use, sexually transmitted diseases, inherited diseases, and serious medical problems.

Family history

You will need to take a family history to determine the health status of the patient's parents, siblings, and other close relatives. This information will help you identify specific risk factors and will serve as a guide for additional diagnostic testing and referral.

Tuberculosis
A family history of tuberculosis places the patient at risk for acquiring the disease.

Pregnancy-induced hypertension (PIH)
The patient is at increased risk if her mother or sisters developed PIH.

Breast cancer
The patient is at increased risk if her mother or any of her mother's female relatives developed the disease. All patients should be taught breast self-examination regardless of family history.

Heart disease
Cardiovascular disease developing in family members before age 50 may signify familial hyperlipidemia. Also, congenital heart defects may be hereditary.

Diabetes
The patient is at increased risk of developing gestational diabetes if family members have developed any form of diabetes.

Epilepsy
This condition is sometimes inherited.

Multiple allergies
These tend to show up in more than one family member.

Multiple gestations
Fraternal twinning is familial (tending to occur among family members).

Congenital anomalies
Congenital anomalies, such as spina bifida, may be familial.

Inherited diseases
Examples include cystic fibrosis and sickle cell anemia.

Mental retardation
Some forms of mental retardation (for example, the mental retardation associated with Down syndrome) may be inherited.

Blindness or deafness (especially from the time of birth)
Such a problem in a family member may indicate an inherited disorder.

Alcoholism
The patient is at increased risk for alcohol abuse if the disease has occurred in her family.

Hepatitis
The patient should be screened for hepatitis if she had direct contact with an infected individual.

Diethylstilbestrol (DES) exposure
The patient is at increased risk for uterine anomalies and vaginal carcinoma if her mother took DES during pregnancy.

Spontaneous abortion
A family history indicating multiple spontaneous abortions may signify chromosomal abnormalities that are not clinically apparent.

Premature labor
The patient may be at increased risk if her mother or sisters experienced preterm labor.

Stillborn infants
A family history of stillborn infants may signify congenital or chromosomal anomalies.

Unexplained childhood deaths
Such deaths may indicate congenital or chromosomal anomalies.

Childhood surgery
Surgeries, such as heart surgery, performed on children are sometimes related to inherited defects.

Early adult deaths
Such deaths may indicate an inherited disorder, such as Marfan's syndrome.

Involuntary infertility
A family history that includes involuntary infertility may indicate chromosomal anomalies.

Patient's history
You will need to obtain the patient's medical and social history to identify specific disorders that may affect the course of pregnancy. Such a history will serve as a guide for additional diagnostic testing and referral and will provide you with an opportunity for patient teaching. Be sure to record the date and method of treatment for those problems your patient may have experienced.

Menstrual history
Determine the patient's age at menarche as well as her current menstrual pattern (before conception), including the frequency of periods, duration, amount of flow, and associated pain.

Kidney disease or recurrent urinary tract infection (UTI)
Patients with such problems should be screened frequently for asymptomatic bacteriuria (ASB). Recurrent UTI is a symptom of diabetes. The stress of pregnancy on renal function may seriously affect patients with preexisting renal disease.

Heart disease
Residual heart damage places the patient at significant risk during pregnancy.

Hypertension
Hypertensive patients are at increased risk for growth-retarded infants and superimposed PIH.

Rheumatic fever
Causing possible permanent damage to heart valves, rheumatic fever may predispose the patient to serious complications related to the normal physiologic changes that occur in the cardiovascular system during pregnancy.

Tuberculosis
Record the date and result of the patient's last tuberculin skin test or chest X-ray.

Sexually transmitted diseases
If the patient has a history of any of the following diseases, she should receive additional screening:
• oral or genital herpes. The patient should report outbreaks during pregnancy.
• syphilis and gonorrhea. The patient should be screened during the initial visit, then later during the third trimester.
• *Chlamydia trachomatis*. The patient should be screened at the initial visit, then later during the third trimester.
• Human papillomavirus (HPV) — virus known to cause venereal warts and genital tract dysplasias.

Patients who are in high-risk groups for human immunodeficiency virus (HIV) should be screened. If the patient's test indicates that she is HIV-positive, she should be advised of the risks to herself and her infant if she continues the pregnancy.

Gynecologic disorders
Recurrent candidal (monilial) infections may be a symptom of diabetes and HIV. Pelvic inflammatory disease predisposes the patient to ectopic pregnancy.

German measles
Be sure to record the age at which your patient was infected or immunized.

Chicken pox
Patients who report no history of varicella should have a varicella titer done. (This identifies the patient who will need varicella-zoster immune globulin within 72 hours of exposure to chicken pox during pregnancy.)

Mental illness or postpartum depression
Postpartum depression tends to recur in subsequent pregnancies.

Diabetes
If the patient is diabetic, she may encounter complications during pregnancy; preventing such complications requires specialized care.

Thyroid dysfunction
Because pregnancy usually affects thyroid function, patients with hyperthyroidism or hypothyroidism require additional laboratory testing during pregnancy.

Thrombophlebitis, presence of varicosities
Pregnancy is a hypercoaguable state. Patients with a history of thrombophlebitis are at risk for recurrence of the disease.

Seizures or epilepsy
If the patient is taking anticonvulsants, she will require careful monitoring of drug levels. Be aware that some anticonvulsants are contraindicated during pregnancy.

Allergies
Note all allergies the patient has to drugs or other substances. If the patient is allergic to iodine, be sure to notify the health care provider as iodine is commonly used to reduce skin bacteria before procedures.

Asthma
Patients taking asthma medication require careful monitoring of drug levels during pregnancy. Some asthma patients seem to notice an improvement in their condition when pregnant, whereas others experience more severe attacks.

Anemia, blood disorders
The added stress of pregnancy on the circulatory system places patients with anemia or blood disorders at risk for complications.

Blood transfusions
If the patient has ever received a blood transfusion, she may be at risk for antibody formation, hepatitis, or HIV infection.

Surgeries (especially those involving the reproductive organs)
If the patient has had any surgical incision into the uterus, she may require delivery by cesarean section.

Serious accidents or injuries (especially to the reproductive tract)
Accidents or injuries may have implications for prenatal care or birth.

Hepatitis
If the patient has had hepatitis B, she must be screened for the chronic carrier state. She also may require liver function tests to rule out residual liver damage following any type of hepatitis infection.

Prescription drugs taken on a regular basis
This information may reveal frequently occurring illnesses or chronic diseases.

Over-the-counter drugs taken frequently
Instruct the patient to avoid all medications unless approved by her doctor. Tell her to avoid aspirin products because they interfere with blood clotting. Ibuprofen also is contraindicated in pregnancy.

Vitamins
Megadoses of certain vitamins can be teratogenic (causing developmental malformations).

Illegal drug use (marijuana, cocaine, or heroin, for example)
If the patient has a history of injectable drug use, she should be screened for hepatitis and HIV infection and should receive specialized care during the pregnancy. The newborn will also require close observation after delivery. Because many women will not admit to drug use, the nurse should be aware of the signs of substance abuse.

Alcohol
Alcohol consumption has been associated with fetal alcohol syndrome. Because no safe level of alcohol consumption during pregnancy has been established, instruct the patient to avoid its use while pregnant.

Tobacco
Tobacco use has been associated with decreased birth weight and prematurity.

History since last menstrual period
The patient's history since the last menstrual period will help you to identify developing complications and factors that may adversely affect the pregnancy. This also provides an opportunity for patient teaching. Be sure to record the date and method of treatment for any problems the patient may have experienced.

Nausea and vomiting
Common throughout the first trimester, nausea and vomiting should be distinguished from a more severe disorder known as hyperemesis gravidarum.

Indigestion
Common during the third trimester, indigestion can be a sign of worsening PIH in a patient with elevated blood pressure.

Constipation
Caution the patient to avoid laxatives.

Headaches
Common during pregnancy, headaches also may be a sign of PIH. If severe, they should be brought to the attention of the health care provider.

Vaginal bleeding
Such bleeding may indicate threatened abortion, abnormal placental location, or vaginal infection.

Vaginal discharge
A possible indication of vaginitis, vaginal discharge should be checked, noting its color and odor and whether it produces itchiness.

Edema
Pedal edema is common during the third trimester. Edema of the face and hands is frequently seen in patients with PIH.

Abdominal pain
Such pain may be associated with certain infections (gynecologic, urinary tract) or premature separation of the placenta. Intermittent pain may actually be preterm labor.

Urinary complaints
Such complaints are a possible symptom of UTI.

Exposure to communicable diseases
Patients who contract diseases such as measles or chicken pox during pregnancy may be at risk for congenital anomalies.

Other illnesses or febrile episodes
Hyperthermia has proved to be teratogenic. Instruct the patient to avoid saunas and hot tubs.

Exposure to radiation
Exposure to X-rays is teratogenic at certain levels.

Obstetric history

During the initial assessment, you'll need to obtain a detailed obstetric history. This information is essential for identifying previous complications that may have an impact on the outcome of the patient's pregnancy.

Date of all previous births or terminations of pregnancy
A history of shortened interpregnancy intervals places the patient at increased risk for certain complications, such as preterm labor and anemia. A patient who is a grand multipara (having given birth to more than five viable fetuses) is at increased risk for complications, such as placenta previa and postpartum hemorrhage.

Duration of each gestation
Recurrent spontaneous abortions may indicate the need for genetic counseling or the presence of a treatable physiologic abnormality, such as a luteal phase defect or an incompetent cervix. Previous preterm births (less than 37 weeks) or postterm births (more than 42 weeks) place the patient at increased risk for recurrence.

Type of birth (spontaneous, forceps, cesarean section)
Difficult forceps deliveries may indicate a degree of cephalopelvic disproportion. Previous cesarean sections may be delivered by repeat cesarean section; however, a trial of labor is recommended for most patients.

Presentation (vertex, breech, other)
Abnormal presentations may recur in subsequent pregnancies.

Anesthesia
Previous reactions to anesthetics may require a change in anesthetic agents.

Episiotomy, lacerations
Extensive lacerations or involvement of the rectal sphincter may indicate previous difficult births.

PREVENTING TOXOPLASMOSIS

If transmitted during pregnancy, toxoplasmosis, an infection caused by a parasite found in raw meat, soil, and cat feces, can cause a newborn to be malformed or to have health-related problems later in life. Patients should be advised to follow these suggestions for preventing toxoplasmosis:
• Cook meat to well done, smoke it, or cure it in salt water.
• Avoid touching the eyes or mucous membranes while handling raw meat.

• Wash hands thoroughly after handling raw meat.
• Wash fruits and vegetables before eating them.
• Keep fruits and vegetables where flies, cockroaches, and other insects cannot touch them.
• Avoid handling things that may be contaminated by cat feces, such as dirt and cat litter boxes.
• Avoid contact with cats that live outdoors.

Maternal complications during the prenatal, intrapartum, or postpartum period
Previous complications, such as PIH, pyelonephritis, and postpartum hemorrhage, may recur. Also, if the patient is Rh-negative, ask whether she received Rh immune globulin.

Newborn birth weight
Newborns weighing more than 8 lb, 13 oz (4,000 g) are considered large for gestational age and may indicate maternal diabetes. The cause for small-for-gestational-age infants should be investigated.

Other information concerning the newborn
Be sure to question the patient concerning the following:
• newborn's sex
• newborn's condition at birth
• whether the newborn was breast- or bottle-fed
• complications that may have occurred in the hospital or after discharge (for example, hypoglycemia, hyperbilirubinemia, or respiratory distress)
• current health and developmental level.

Additional information
Obtain the following information:

Date of last tetanus vaccination
If the vaccination was more than 10 years ago, the patient can be vaccinated after the first trimester.

Pets
If the patient has a cat, caution her about the transmission of toxoplasmosis. All patients should receive specific preventive instructions regarding toxoplasmosis (see *Preventing toxoplasmosis*).

Birth control used at time of conception
Oral contraceptives have been implicated in a small increase in birth defects. Although researchers haven't proved an association between spermicidal creams and jellies and birth defects, successful lawsuits have been brought against the manufacturers of such products.

PREVENTING AND TREATING MORNING SICKNESS WITHOUT DRUGS

Morning sickness, the term applied to the nausea and vomiting that often occur during the early months of pregnancy, can occur any time of the day or night. Usually, it disappears after about the 3rd month.

Early in pregnancy, the ovaries produce increased amounts of estrogen and progesterone. Because of the increasing levels of these hormones, the stomach's secretory cells increase production of gastric juices. Simultaneously, the bowel slows down in its ability to empty the stomach contents, which causes a feeling of nausea and, sometimes, vomiting.

Advise the patient to try any of the following suggestions:

To prevent morning sickness
• Before getting out of bed in the morning, eat a piece of bread or a few crackers (put them close to your bed the night before).
• Get out of bed slowly; avoid sudden movements.
• Eat foods high in protein, such as eggs, cheese, nuts, and meats as well as fruits and fruit juices. This helps prevent low blood glucose levels, which also can cause nausea.
• Drink soups and other liquids between, instead of with, meals.
• Avoid greasy or fried foods, which are hard to digest.
• Avoid spicy or heavily seasoned foods.

To treat morning sickness
• Sip soda water (carbonated water) at the onset of nausea.
• Get plenty of fresh air (take a walk, sleep with a window open).
• Take deep breaths.
• Drink spearmint, raspberry leaf, or peppermint tea.
• Try any of the prevention tips listed above.
Note: If your patient's vomiting persists or if it becomes difficult for her to retain food or liquids, advise her to contact her health care provider. Tell her to avoid using over-the counter antinausea medications, unless prescribed by the health care provider.

Last menstrual period
Knowing this information will help to determine the patient's expected date of confinement (EDC), or delivery date. To do so, count back 3 months from the first day of her last menstrual period and add 7 days (Nägele's rule).

First fetal movement (quickening)
Most multiparous women feel quickening around 16 to 18 weeks of pregnancy, most primigravidas at about 18 to 20 weeks.

Nutritional assessment

The patient's nutritional level during pregnancy will greatly affect the pregnancy's outcome. An average of 300 extra calories per day are required during pregnancy. Use the following information to help the patient plan an adequate prenatal diet:

24-hour diet recall
Instruct the patient to record everything that she eats for a typical day. This can serve as a guide for nutritional counseling.

Number of meals per day
Regular meals spaced throughout the day plus a bedtime snack will prevent the development of ketosis.

Nausea and vomiting
Normal nausea and vomiting that occurs during the early months of pregnancy can be treated with a dry diet (see *Preventing and treating morning sickness without drugs* for additional suggestions).

RECOMMENDED DIETARY ALLOWANCES[a]

		Pregnant	Breast-feeding (First 6 months)	Breast-feeding (Second 6 months)
	Protein (g)	60.0	65.0	62.0
Fat-soluble vitamins	Vitamin A (μg RE)[b]	800.0	1,300.0	1,200.0
	Vitamin D (μg)[c]	10.0	10.0	10.0
	Vitamin E (mg α-TE)[d]	10.0	12.0	11.0
	Vitamin K (μg)	65.0	65.0	65.0
Water-soluble vitamins	Vitamin C (mg)	70.0	95.0	90.0
	Folate (μg)	400.0	280.0	260.0
	Niacin (mg NE)[e]	17.0	20.0	20.0
	Riboflavin (mg)	1.6	1.8	1.7
	Thiamin (mg)	1.5	1.6	1.6
	Vitamin B_6 (mg)	2.2	2.1	2.1
	Vitamin B_{12} (μg)	2.2	2.6	2.6
Minerals	Calcium (mg)	1,200.0	1,200.0	1,200.0
	Phosphorus (mg)	1,200.0	1,200.0	1,200.0
	Iodine (μg)	175.0	200.0	200.0
	Iron (mg)	30.0	15.0	15.0
	Magnesium (mg)	300.0	355.0	340.0
	Zinc (mg)	15.0	19.0	16.0
	Selenium (μg)	65.0	75.0	75.0

a. The allowances, expressed as average daily intakes over time, are intended to provide for individual variations among most normal persons as they live in the United States under usual environmental stresses. Because there is less information on which to base allowances, the ranges of recommended adult intake of the vitamins biotin and pantothenic acid are 30 μg to 100 μg and 4 to 7 mg, respectively. Diets should be based on a variety of common foods in order to provide other nutrients for which human requirements have been less well defined.
b. Retinol equivalents. 1 retinol equivalent = 1 μg retinol or 6 μg beta carotene.
c. As cholecalciferol, 10 μg cholecalciferol = 400 IU vitamin D.
d. Alpha-tocopherol equivalents (α-TE). 1 mg d-α-tocopherol = 1 α-TE.
e. 1 NE (niacin equivalent) is equal to 1 mg of niacin or 60 mg of dietary tryptophan.

Adapted with permission from *Recommended Dietary Allowances*, 10th ed. © 1989 by the National Academy of Sciences, National Academy Press, Washington, D.C.

DAILY FOOD PATTERN FOR PREGNANCY

Food	Amount
Milk, nonfat or low -fat; yogurt; and cheese	3 to 4 cups
Meat (lean), poultry, fish, egg	2 servings (total of 4 to 6 oz)
Vegetables, cooked or raw dark green or yellow, starchy, including potatoes, dried peas, and beans; all others	3 to 5 servings
Whole-grain and enriched breads and cereals	7 or more servings
Fats and sweets	In moderate amounts

Food allergies
Allergy to milk may place the patient at risk for calcium deficiency.

Cravings for specific foods or other substances
Pica refers to the regular and excessive ingestion of nonfood items (such as clay or laundry starch) or foods with limited nutritional value (such as ice).

Specific cultural, religious, or personal dietary restrictions
Vegetarian diets may be deficient in some vitamins and nutrients; religious practices of fasting may lead to ketosis; and culturally determined eating patterns may affect nutritional status (for example, Blacks tend to consume a high-fat diet; Asians favor low-protein diets).

Vitamin and iron supplements
Such supplements are recommended to meet the increased demands of pregnancy. To reduce the frequency of neural tube defects, all pregnant women should consume 0.4 mg of folic acid per day. Ideally, this supplementation should begin prior to conception. (See *Recommended dietary allowances,* page 11, and *Daily food pattern for pregnancy,* above).

Performing the physical examination
To determine the patient's general state of health and detect any deviations from normal, a complete physical examination should be performed. Confirming the pregnancy and establishing the length of gestation are important components of the physical examination. The examination should begin with recording the following:

Vital signs
Taking vital signs includes noting the patient's temperature, pulse rate, respirations, and blood pressure. During pregnancy, the patient's pulse rate increases by 15 to 20 beats/minute; the respiratory rate increases by about 2 respirations/minute. Blood pressure should be taken with the patient in a sitting position; the first trimester reading, a more accurate measure of the patient's normal blood pressure, will be used as the baseline measurement throughout the pregnancy. Keep in mind the following information when comparing baseline measurements to those taken later in the pregnancy:
• Second-trimester systolic and diastolic rates should decrease by 5 to 10 mm Hg. Patients who do not demonstrate this decrease are at risk for PIH.
• Third-trimester blood pressure measurements should return to baseline levels.
• Any increase of 30 mm Hg systolic or 15 mm Hg diastolic over the patient's prepregnant or early first trimester blood pressure is considered abnormal.

Weight
During pregnancy, a woman of normal prepregnant weight should gain 25-35 lb (11.3-15.9 kg); underweight women, 28-40 lb (12.7-18.2 kg); and overweight women, 15-25 lb (6.8-11.3 kg). Note the following:
• During the first trimester, a total gain of 3 lb (1.4 kg) is recommended.
• After the first trimester, patients normally gain ¾ to 1 lb (340 to 454 g) per week.
• A weight gain of more than 2 lb (0.9 kg) per week, or more than 6 lb (2.7 kg) per month, is considered abnormal and may indicate excessive fluid retention.
• Patients weighing less than 100 lb (45.4 kg) or more than 200 lb (90.8 kg) at the onset of pregnancy are at increased risk for complications.

Height
Patients who are less than 5' (1.5 m) tall are considered to be at risk for preterm labor.

Skin
Some normal physiologic changes occur during pregnancy; note any of the following:
• hyperpigmentation (chloasma [mask of pregnancy], linea nigra, nevi, or darkening of nipples), resulting from increased melanocyte activity
• striae gravidarum (stretch marks) caused by separations within the connective tissue over areas of maximum stretch
• vascular spiders on the neck, thorax, face, or arms
• palmar erythema (caused by a high-estrogen state)
• increased sweat and sebaceous gland activity.

Hair
The patient's hair should be examined for pediculosis (head lice).

Eyes
The patient's sclerae should be examined for jaundice. Xanthelasma (fatty deposits around the eyes) may indicate familial hyperlipidemia.

Ears
The ear canals and tympanic membranes should be examined for signs of infection or abnormalities.

Mouth
The gums may be swollen or may bleed easily, resulting from a high-estrogen state. Ptyalism (excessive salivation) also may occur. Dental hygiene and the presence of caries should be noted.

Neck
The patient's neck should be examined for enlarged lymph nodes; the thyroid gland, for size and the presence of masses. (most patients' thyroid glands enlarge bilaterally as a result of increased glandular activity and may be palpable).

Heart
During pregnancy, the heart enlarges slightly and becomes displaced upward and to the left. In 95% of all pregnant patients, systolic murmurs can be heard as a result of increased blood volume.

Chest
Breath sounds, auscultated bilaterally, should be clear.

Breasts
During pregnancy, the breasts increase in size and vascularity. Colostrum may be present as early as the 16th week of pregnancy. Advise the patient that she should continue monthly breast self-examinations throughout the pregnancy and that, if she has flat or inverted nipples, she will require additional preparation for breast-feeding (see *Preparing for breast-feeding*).

Abdomen
The patient's abdomen should be examined for enlargement of the liver and spleen; they should not be palpable. The height of the fundus is measured (see *Measuring fundal height,* page 16). Fetal heart tones are auscultated; they should be audible with a Doppler probe at 10 to 12 weeks or with a fetoscope at 18 to 20 weeks.

Back
The patient's back is examined for costovertebral angle tenderness (CVAT), which may indicate pyelonephritis. Also, check for scoliosis.

Extremities
The patient's extremities are examined for varicosities and edema of the feet (a normal finding late in pregnancy). Deep tendon reflexes should be checked; if the patient is hyperreflexic (3 + or

PREPARING FOR BREAST-FEEDING

The woman who is interested in breast-feeding should be acquainted with pertinent information early in her pregnancy. The earlier she receives information, the more likely she will breast-feed successfully for a substantial period of time. The majority of preparation for breast-feeding will be done in the last trimester; however, the woman should be examined during the initial physical exam to determine if she has flat or inverted nipples, which may require additional preparation for successful breast-feeding. In addition, the nurse should inform the woman early in pregnancy about how to care for her breasts so that future problems can be avoided.

The woman should be instructed to do the following:
• Avoid washing the nipple and areola with soap (removes the skin oils and interferes with the natural acid-alkaline balance)
• Avoid scrubbing nipples (wears away natural oils, causing the skin to dry and crack) and drying or hardening agents such as tincture of benzoin, witch hazel, and pHisoHex
• Remove plastic liners in nursing bras or nursing pads (produce a warm, moist environment for breeding bacteria)
• Use no additional lubricants.

During the third trimester, the mother should begin routine nipple preparation. Additional layers of keratin can be produced by the skin of the nipples and areola with proper preparation. Techniques for building keratin include the following:
• Exposure to air and sunlight
• Nipple tug and roll
• Breast massage

• Stimulation during sexual activity.

Because any type of nipple stimulation can produce uterine activity as a result of the release of oxytocin from the posterior pituitary, women with a history of preterm labor and those at risk for developing this complication during pregnancy (such as twins) should consult with their health care provider prior to starting nipple preparation.

In the past, many sources advised the pregnant woman to express colostrum prenatally. Removal of colostrum is not advisable because it presents a possible hazard of inducing labor. Because colostrum acts as a barrier to bacteria and viruses, removing it also could leave the breast susceptible to infection. It also is not known if colostrum is continually produced with consistent quantities of each component, thus prenatal removal may deprive the infant of this essential food both in terms of quantity and quality.

Nipple correction

If the mother has flat or inverted nipples, she will need additional preparation during the third trimester to help correct this problem. Milk cups (breast shields) worn inside the bra will exert gentle pressure around the nipple making the skin more pliable and the nipple easier to grasp. The Hoffman technique involves gentle pulling on opposite sides of the areola, which will help the nipple to protrude. Once the nipple has become protractile enough to grasp, the nipple tug and roll can be added to the routine.

4+), check for clonus. Hyperreflexia and the presence of clonus are associated with PIH.

Pelvic area

An examination of the patient's external genitalia should include the following:
• pattern of hair growth
• lesions that may indicate sexually transmitted disease (herpes, condyloma acuminatum)
• varicosities of the vulva or perineum
• vaginal outlet (relaxed or constricted)
• perineum length and presence of old scars
• hemorrhoids and sphincter control

An examination of the internal structures usually includes:
• vaginal lesions or prolapse

MEASURING FUNDAL HEIGHT

By estimating your patient's uterine size, you can evaluate the fetus' gestational age by measuring fundal height. Between weeks 18 and 32 of pregnancy, the fundal height in centimeters equals the fetus's age in weeks. For example, if your patient is at 24 weeks, her fundal height should be about 24 cm. Remember, though, that fundal height measurements taken late in pregnancy may not be accurate; fetal weight variations and engagement can distort your reading.

To measure fundal height, follow these steps. With your patient in a supine position, place the end of a tape measure at the level of her symphysis pubis. Stretch the tape to the top of the uterine fundus. Record this measurement. Another method of determining fundal height involves using three landmarks: the symphysis pubis, the umbilicus, and the xiphoid process. At 16 weeks, the fundus can be found halfway between the symphysis pubis and the umbilicus. At 20 to 22 weeks, the fundus is at the umbilicus. At 36 weeks, the fundus is at the xiphoid process.

Remember: such factors as a full bladder, amniotic fluid volume, or obesity may affect fundal height measurement.

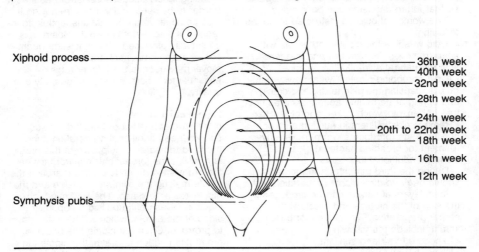

Xiphoid process

36th week
40th week
32nd week
28th week
24th week
20th to 22nd week
18th week
16th week
12th week

Symphysis pubis

• abnormal discharge (color, odor, consistency)
• cervix (bleeding, lesions, lacerations, position, consistency, dilatation, effacement)
• uterus (consistency, shape, size)
• adnexa (early in pregnancy, this should be examined to rule out masses; after 12 weeks, it will not be palpable as a pelvic structure because of uterine growth)
• size of bony pelvis (gross measurement by clinical pelvimetry)
• rectum (lesions, hemorrhoids, sphincter control).

Laboratory tests in the prenatal period

Laboratory tests will vary from one setting to another, depending on the risk factors identified in the individual patient's prenatal history and physical examination. Below is a listing of some commonly ordered tests (see Section 3 for a list of other tests).

Blood type, Rh factor, irregular antibodies
If the patient is Rh-negative and has a negative antibody screen, she will need a repeat antibody screen at week 28 and should receive Rh immune globulin if the antibody screen is negative. The presence of antibodies known to cause hemolytic disease of the newborn (the D factor of the Rh group and antigens of the Lewis, Kell, Duffy, and Kidd groups) requires specialized care during the prenatal period.

Rubella titer
If the patient has a negative titer, indicating susceptibility to the rubella virus, ensure that she receives the proper immunization postpartum.

Hemoglobin and hematocrit levels
Expect the patient's hemoglobin and hematocrit levels to drop during gestation as a result of increased plasma volume. A rise in the hematocrit level may indicate the development of PIH, whereas a drop in hemoglobin (below 10 g/dl) and hematocrit (below 30%) levels indicates anemia. Hemoglobin and hematocrit levels are repeated during the second and third trimesters.

Syphilis screening (Venereal Disease Research Laboratory [VDRL] test, rapid plasma reagin test [RPR])
Patients should be tested for syphilis at the initial visit and during the third trimester if in a high-risk group.

HIV
All patients should be offered screening. Informed consent and counseling is necessary prior to testing.

Sickle cell screening
This test is indicated for patients at risk for sickle cell disease (Blacks or those of Mediterranean ancestry). A positive test indicates a need for further screening using hemoglobin electrophoresis.

Hepatitis B surface antigen
The Centers for Disease Control recently recommended that all women be screened for hepatitis B. However, if selected screening is done, the following groups should be included:
• patients who were born in Asia, Africa, Haiti, or the Pacific Basin as well as those of Inuit descent
• health care workers who have been exposed to blood or blood products
• workers in institutions for the mentally retarded
• patients with previously undiagnosed jaundice or chronic liver disease
• parenteral drug abusers
• patients with tatoos
• patients with a history of blood transfusions
• patients with a history of multiple episodes of sexually transmitted disease

• patients who have been previously rejected as blood donors
• patients with a history of dialysis or renal transplantation
• patients from households having hepatitis B-infected members
or hemodialysis patients.

Maternal serum alpha-fetoprotein screening (MSAFP)
MSAFP (MSAFP plus, triscreen, triplescreen) is offered to all patients. Maternal blood is drawn and examined for alpha-fetoprotein, HCG, and estriol to detect neural tube defects and Down
syndrome. (See alpha-fetoprotein, section 3).

Tuberculin skin test
This test should be performed only if all past skin tests have
been negative. A positive skin test indicates the need for a chest
X-ray (using an abdominal shield) to rule out active disease.
Converters may be referred after delivery for isoniazid prophy-
laxis.

Papanicolaou smear
A Papanicolaou (Pap) smear is done during the initial prenatal
examination to screen for cervical intraepithelial neoplasia.

Gonorrhea culture
This screening test should be repeated during the third trimester
in high-risk patients.

Chlamydia culture
Screening for *Chlamydia* is indicated if the patient is in a high-
risk group or infants from previous pregnancies have developed
neonatal conjunctivitis or pneumonia.

Group B streptococcal culture
Vaginal cultures for group B streptococci may be routine or for
patients in high-risk groups.

Urinalysis and urine culture
Obtain a urine specimen for glucose and protein analyses at every visit; periodic screening for infection is indicated for patients
at risk. Keep in mind the following information:
• Glycosuria, a common result of decreased renal threshold in
pregnancy, may indicate diabetes if it persists.
• Test results indicating a trace or a 1+ level of proteinuria are
frequently the result of contamination; levels of 2+ to 4+ may
indicate infection or PIH.
• Ketonuria may result from insufficient food intake or vomiting.
• White blood cells and bacteria in a clean-catch specimen may
indicate infection.

Home care guidelines
• Encourage some type of regular exercise for all women.
• Common discomforts often can be managed by self-care mea-
sures.

IDENTIFYING DANGER SIGNS OF PREGNANCY

If your patient develops any of the following signs or symptoms, instruct her to notify the health care provider immediately.

Sign or symptom	Possible indication
Dyspnea	Impending cardiac decompensation, premature separation of the placenta, excessive amniotic fluid accumulation, or pulmonary embolus
Persistent or recurring headache	Pregnancy-induced hypertension
Persistent nausea and vomiting	Hyperemesis gravidarum or systemic infection
Vision changes (flashing lights, dots before eyes, dimming or blurring of vision)	Pregnancy-induced hypertension
Dizziness when not supine	Hypoglycemia, anemia, or cardiac arrhythmias
Abdominal pain	Ectopic pregnancy, abruptio placentae, or uterine rupture
Edema of the face and hands	Pregnancy-induced hypertension
No fetal movements for 8 hours or a significant decrease from one day to the next	Fetal distress or death
Vaginal bleeding	Placenta previa, abruptio placentae, or spontaneous abortion
Sudden escape of fluid from the vagina	Premature rupture of membranes
Burning or pain on urination	Urinary tract infection or pyelonephritis
Unusual skin rashes or sores	Infectious diseases
Signs of labor occurring more than 3 weeks before estimated date of confinement	Premature labor

- Make sure the patient receives a list of danger signs and symptoms. Instruct her to notify her health care provider immediately if any occur and make sure she receives instructions on how to reach the health care provider when the office or clinic is closed (see *Identifying danger signs of pregnancy*).
- Instruct the patient in the proper use of seatbelts.

☐ Subsequent prenatal visits

Regular prenatal visits are essential to ensure consistent, quality care. Unless the patient has a particular problem that warrants a

PERFORMING LEOPOLD'S MANEUVERS

If your patient is at least 28 weeks pregnant, use the four Leopold's maneuvers to determine fetal position. During late pregnancy, you can also use them to identify fetal presentation and anticipate labor and delivery complications.

As a rule, you can accurately assess fetal position after the 28th week because the uterine and abdominal muscles are stretched and thinned. But you may have trouble assessing fetal position if the patient has hydramnios, she's very obese, she's carrying

1. The *first maneuver* will determine which part of the fetus is in the fundus. First, stand beside the table and face your patient. Place your palms at each side of her upper abdomen. Curl your fingers around the fundus. If the head is in the fundus, you'll feel a hard, round, movable object. The buttocks are more difficult to move: they'll feel soft and have an irregular shape.

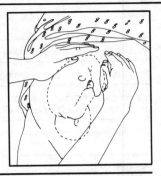

2. For the *second maneuver*, move your hands downward over each side of your patient's abdomen, applying firm, even pressure. On one side of her abdomen, you should feel the fetus' back—a smooth, hard surface that offers resistance as you press inward. On the opposite side, you may feel irregular knobs or lumps; these are the fetus's hands, feet, elbows and knees.

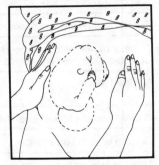

special visit, the recommended frequency of visits is once a month until the 28th week, then once every 2 weeks until the 36th week, then once a week until birth.

General assessment

During subsequent visits, the patient assessment should include the following:
• finding out about the patient's general well-being, complaints, and problems
• weighing the patient; compare this weight to the last weight obtained and assess any gain to date as well as the pattern of weight gain
• checking for edema of the feet, hands and face
• obtaining a urine specimen for glucose and protein analyses; check the urine for ketones if the patient has failed to gain or has lost weight

more than one fetus, the fetus is unusually small, a tumor or other unusual growth is present in the uterus, or the placenta's placement obstructs palpation.

Before you begin, ask the patient to empty her bladder so you won't confuse it with the fetus' head. Also, warm your hands before starting, and apply them with firm but gentle pressure. Otherwise, the patient's muscles may contract, impairing your ability to assess fetal position.

3. For the *third maneuver*, spread the thumb and fingers of one hand as wide as possible. Place your hand just above your patient's symphysis pubis. Then, bring your thumb and fingers together. As you do, grasp the part of the fetus that's between them: either the head or buttocks. You'll do this to confirm the fetal position you determined in the first maneuver.

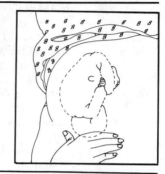

4. Use the *fourth maneuver* in late stages of pregnancy to determine how far the fetus has descended into the pelvic inlet. Turn and face your patient's feet and place your hands on the sides of her lower abdomen, close to midline. Slide your hands downward and press inward. If you've already determined that the fetus' buttocks are in the fundus, then feel for the head. If you can't feel it, then it has probably descended.

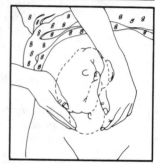

- taking blood pressure measurements
- determining the frequency and pattern of fetal activity
- examining the patient's abdomen by:
  - measuring fundal height
  - auscultating the fetal heart rate
  - performing Leopold's maneuvers to determine position and presentation after 28 weeks' gestation (see *Performing Leopold's maneuvers*)
- performing additional tests, as ordered
- assessing the patient's educational needs
- assessing the patient's emotional adjustment to pregnancy and approaching parenthood.

☐ Nursing diagnoses and interventions (prenatal)

Here is a listing of some of the nursing diagnoses and interventions frequently associated with the normal prenatal period.

Nursing diagnosis

Altered Nutrition: Less Than Body Requirements related to nausea and vomiting, self-imposed caloric restriction, or inadequate financial resources
Desired outcome: Patient will experience a normal weight gain during pregnancy.

Nursing interventions and rationales

1. Perform a nutritional assessment early in pregnancy.
Rationale: This will identify areas of concern and allow for intervention before complications occur.
2. Provide counseling regarding normal nutritional alterations necessary during pregnancy.
Rationale: Many women are unaware of dietary needs during pregnancy.
3. Refer the patient to additional sources of nutrition when necessary.
Rationale: A government-supported supplement program (WIC) is available for pregnant women in need.
4. Instruct the patient to follow a dry diet if nausea or vomiting is present during the first trimester.
Rationale: A dry diet is often successful in treating normal morning sickness.

Nursing diagnosis

Pain related to heartburn caused by pressure on the cardiac sphincter from the expanding uterus
Desired outcome: Patient will obtain relief from heartburn discomfort through dietary changes or medication.

Nursing interventions and rationales

1. Advise the patient to decrease the amount of fat in her diet.
Rationale: Fatty foods tend to aggravate heartburn.
2. Suggest that the patient avoid coffee and cigarettes.
Rationale: These products stimulate acid secretion in the stomach and irritate the mucosa.
3. Recommend that the patient eat several small meals (five or six) per day.
Rationale: Smaller meals do not overfill the stomach; they decrease the pressure against the cardiac sphincter.
4. Caution the patient to avoid lying down after meals.
Rationale: The supine position pushes food against the cardiac sphincter.
5. Propose the use of antacids, as recommended by the health care provider.
Rationale: These products neutralize the acids in the stomach, which are irritating. Antacids with an aluminum or magnesium base are recommended. Instruct the patient to avoid antacids

that are high in sodium when using such products.
6. Report any persistent, severe heartburn to the health care provider.
Rationale: Heartburn can be a symptom of edema of the liver capsule in severe PIH.

Nursing diagnosis
Altered Urinary Elimination related to physiologic changes during pregnancy
Desired outcome: Patient will have no complications of the genitourinary or lower gastrointestinal tract during pregnancy.

Nursing interventions and rationales
1. Advise the patient that frequency of urination is common during the first and third trimesters.
Rationale: Pressure of the uterus on the bladder causes frequent desire to urinate.
2. Instruct the patient to report all flank pain, burning, and pain with urination.
Rationale: Pregnant patients are at increased risk for urinary tract infections caused by normal changes in the genitourinary tract during pregnancy.

Nursing diagnosis
Constipation related to normal physiologic changes during pregnancy
Desired outcome: Patient will maintain a normal bowel pattern during pregnancy.

Nursing interventions and rationales
1. Counsel the patient to increase her intake of fluids, fruits, vegetables, and bran products.
Rationale: Eating these foods prevents constipation.
2. Instruct the patient to use stool softeners, as ordered, but to avoid harsh laxatives and mineral oil.
Rationale: Stool softeners may be helpful, as ordered; however, harsh laxatives may precipitate uterine activity and should not be used. Mineral oil prevents absorption of fat-soluble vitamins.

Nursing diagnosis
High Risk for Infection of the Vagina related to increased vaginal secretions during pregnancy
Desired outcome: Patient will have no complications from vaginal infections during gestation.

Nursing interventions and rationales
1. Caution the patient to avoid douching.

Rationale: Douching disturbs the normal flora of the vagina and may predispose the patient to infections.

2. Advise the patient to avoid feminine hygiene sprays.
Rationale: Use of such products can cause severe perineal irritations.

3. Notify the health care provider if abnormal symptoms (such as itching, foul odor, or profuse discharge) occur.
Rationale: Untreated infections may be associated with preterm labor, premature rupture of the membranes, and infections in the newborn.

Nursing diagnosis
Fear related to the possibility of having an abnormal child
Desired outcome: Patient will be screened appropriately during pregnancy and referred for further testing or counseling, as necessary.

Nursing interventions and rationales
1. Obtain a thorough family and patient history to identify the need for genetic counseling.
Rationale: Such a history will help identify patients at risk for genetic defects.

2. Monitor the pregnancy's progress carefully.
Rationale: Delayed fetal growth, polyhydramnios, or abnormal findings on ultrasound may indicate the presence of anomalies.

3. Provide emotional support if the patient is referred for further evaluation.
Rationale: The waiting period for test results causes extreme anxiety. The possibility of having an abnormal child may threaten the couple's self-esteem.

Nursing diagnosis
High Risk for Injury related to complications of pregnancy
Desired outcome: Patient will have no preventable complications during pregnancy.

Nursing interventions and rationales
1. Instruct the patient about what danger signs to watch for during pregnancy.
Rationale: Early recognition of a problem by the patient in many cases will help minimize complications.

2. Monitor the patient closely for deviations from the normal progress of pregnancy.
Rationale: Early recognition of signs of complications allows for prompt intervention.

3. Assure the patient that someone will be available to listen to her reports of problems or to answer her questions.
Rationale: Patients need to feel comfortable when calling to report symptoms and to ask questions.

Nursing diagnosis

Knowledge Deficit related to normal changes during pregnancy, fetal growth and development, the effect of pregnancy on the family, and diet restrictions or changes during pregnancy

Desired outcome: Patient will become properly educated during pregnancy in those areas, both physical and psychological, which are necessary to achieve a healthy pregnancy.

Nursing interventions and rationales

1. Discuss with the patient her knowledge about pregnancy and parenthood as well as her future educational needs.

Rationale: This discussion will provide information that can be used to plan an educational program for the patient.

2. Refer the patient to educational programs provided by local hospitals and other institutions or organizations.

Rationale: Excellent prenatal programs are available in most communities.

3. Provide the patient with an opportunity to ask questions and to take part in educational programs during visits.

Rationale: Patients may feel more comfortable asking questions in a private setting.

4. Provide written educational materials in the office setting.

Rationale: Because patients may feel embarrassed about asking certain questions, providing written materials ensures another means of patient teaching.

5. Include the patient's partner in all prenatal visits and educational sessions.

Rationale: Including the patient's partner will help prepare him for parenthood. It also will help the baby's father to feel more a part of the progress of the pregnancy.

☐ Assessment during labor and delivery

Your patient will probably come to the labor and delivery unit when one of the following has occurred:

• She is experiencing a pattern of increasingly intense uterine contractions.

• The membranes are leaking or have ruptured.

• She is experiencing certain symptoms that are of concern to her or to the health care provider.

Regardless of the reason, you'll need to make an initial assessment and collect the necessary information so that the doctor or nurse midwife can establish a plan of care for the patient.

General admission information

After reviewing the prenatal record, note the following patient information:

- age (Teenagers and those over age 35 are at increased risk for certain complications.)
- expected date of confinement (Determine whether the pregnancy is term, preterm, or postdate; preterm and postdate may have a significant impact on labor and delivery.)
- laboratory test results, including:
  - blood type, Rh factor, antibody screen
  - serology for syphilis
  - last hemoglobin and hematocrit levels
  - gonorrhea culture
  - HIV
  - hepatitis B surface antigen
  - any other significant laboratory tests
- prenatal complications
- allergies
- history of herpes infection.

Nursing history

After obtaining the general patient information, proceed with taking the patient's nursing history. Include the following information in your notes.

Contractions

Record the time of onset of contractions, their frequency and duration, and the degree of discomfort they cause the patient.

Status of the membranes

If the patient is not at term or in labor, but the membranes have ruptured, avoid performing a vaginal examination, which could introduce infection. However, be sure to note the time of rupture, because prolonged rupture of membranes (ROM) is associated with infection.

Bleeding

Distinguish between bleeding and normal show. If the patient is bleeding, do not perform a vaginal examination until placenta previa has been ruled out.

Fetal activity

Monitoring fetal activity is an indirect measure of fetal well-being.

Current medications

Carefully note any medications the patient is currently taking; this information may be essential to the health care provider.

Last food ingested

Record what the patient ate and when. Because stomach emptying time slows during labor, food may be retained in the stomach, causing nausea and vomiting.

Analgesia or anesthesia

Note what type of analgesia or anesthesia has been planned.

Preparation for childbirth

Ask the patient about her preparations for childbirth, including:

- prenatal classes attended
- who will be her support person during labor
- the pediatrician's name
- her decision on how the baby will be fed.

Physical assessment

After recording the nursing history, begin the physical assessment, including the following data:

Vital signs

When taking vital sign measurements, note the patient's:
- temperature. The patient's temperature should be within normal limits; elevation may indicate dehydration or infection.
- pulse rate. A pulse rate of more than 100 beats/minute suggests dehydration, exhaustion, infection, or blood loss.
- respirations. The respiration rate should be within normal limits.
- blood pressure. The blood pressure measurement should be taken between contractions, as pressures taken during contractions may be slightly increased.

Fetal evaluation

To assess the condition of the fetus:
- perform Leopold's maneuvers to determine position, presentation, and engagement
- check the fetal heart rate (check the rate before, during, and after a contraction or place the patient on an external fetal monitor; 120 to 160 beats/minute is considered the normal range).

Evaluation of contractions

Assess the frequency, duration, and intensity of contractions by palpation and the use of an electronic monitor, if available.

Pelvic examination

To determine the membrane status, perform a sterile speculum examination, including the following:
- a nitrazine test, in which pH paper turns blue in presence of alkaline amniotic fluid (see "Nitrazine test" in Section 3)
- a fern test, in which amniotic fluid that has dried on a glass slide appears as a cluster of fern leaves under the microscope (see "Fern test" in Section 3)
- noting the color of amniotic fluid if the membranes have ruptured; meconium-stained fluid can be an indication of fetal distress.

Vaginal examination

Check for the following:
- cervical dilatation and effacement
- fetal presentation and position
- station of the presenting part
- degree of molding of the fetal head; increased molding may indicate cephalopelvic disproportion.

Laboratory data

Note the following laboratory results in the patient's record:
• urinalysis for protein and ketone levels
• hemoglobin and hematocrit levels (may be falsely elevated because of dehydration)
• white blood cell count (usually elevated during labor).

Ongoing assessment during labor

During labor, you'll need to assess the patient's condition frequently. Be sure to check the following maternal and fetal parameters:

Maternal vital signs
Vital sign measurements should include:
• temperature (taken every 4 hours until membranes rupture, then every 2 hours)
• pulse and respirations (taken every 4 hours)
• blood pressure (taken every hour; however, if the patient has PIH or if epidural anesthesia is in use, blood pressure should be recorded every 15 minutes).

Fetal heart rate
Note the following information about measuring fetal heart rate.
• Most institutions use electronic fetal monitoring, which provides a continuous readout of the fetal heart rate (see "Fetal monitoring" in Section 3).
• Auscultation (performed by counting for a full minute and listening through a contraction) should be performed once every hour during early labor, once every ½ hour during active labor, and after each contraction in the second stage of labor.

Timing of contractions
Be sure to measure the frequency, duration, and intensity of contractions by palpation or by use of an electronic monitor, if available. The average frequency of contractions is once every 10 minutes during early labor to once every 2 or 3 minutes in the second stage of labor.

Duration of contractions
Durations of 30 seconds during early labor and 60 to 90 seconds during the second stage are considered normal. Report any contraction lasting longer than 90 seconds to the health care provider. Keep in mind that the patient must have adequate rest between contractions to prevent maternal exhaustion, fetal distress, and uterine rupture.

Intensity of contractions
Gauge intensity as mild, moderate, or strong according to how far you are able to indent the fundus with your fingertips — or more accurately, by use of an internal pressure catheter inserted by the health care provider.

Rupture of the membranes

Prolonged rupture of the membranes is associated with the development of infection. When the membranes rupture, be sure to include the following in your assessment:
- Observe the color of the amniotic fluid. Meconium-stained fluid may be a sign of fetal distress.
- Note any odor. Foul-smelling fluid is associated with infection.
- Consider the amount of fluid. Scant amounts may indicate a growth-retarded fetus, post-date pregnancy, or fetal anomaly, whereas excessive amounts may indicate other fetal anomalies, diabetes, or subsequent development of abruptio placentae.
- Measure the fetal heart rate. If the presenting part does not fill the pelvic inlet, the cord may wash down with the fluid, causing compression of the vessels that supply the fetus with oxygen (prolapsed cord). By auscultating the fetal heart rate after rupture of membranes, you can determine if this has occurred.

Vaginal examination

Assess the patient for dilatation, effacement, station, and degree of molding of the fetal head. Indications for vaginal examination include the following:
- rupturing of the membranes (spontaneous or artificial)
- a change in the monitor tracing of the fetal heart rate
- the patient's urge to push
- pain medication administration (examination occurs before administration)
- need for reassessment because labor is not proceeding at a normal rate

Intake and output

During labor, the patient is given nothing by mouth; however, sometimes ice or clear fluids are permitted in some institutions. Remember to do the following:
- Monitor the patient's I.V. fluids.
- Encourage the patient to void every 2 hours.
- Check the patient's bladder for distention; because of anesthesia or the pressure created by the presenting part, the patient may be unaware of the need to void.

Position during labor

The patient's position during labor is determined by the patient's individual preference, the monitoring equipment used, and the presence of complications. Avoid placing the patient in the dorsal recumbent position to prevent the development of vena cava syndrome; the weight of the gravid uterus compresses the ascending vena cava, causing decreased cardiac output and hypotension.

Psychological factors

When assessing the patient's psychological response to labor, remember to:
- appraise the patient's need for additional emotional support

• evaluate the support person's ability to help the patient cope with labor

• assess the patient's need for medication to facilitate the physical and emotional process of labor (see "Epidural block" in Section 3).

☐ Nursing diagnoses and interventions (normal labor and delivery)

Below is a listing of the nursing diagnoses and interventions frequently associated with normal labor and delivery.

Nursing diagnosis

Pain related to uterine contractions and cervical dilation
Desired outcome: Patient will be able to cope with the discomfort of labor.

Nursing interventions and rationales

1. Assess the patient's preparation for labor.
Rationale: Patients who have attended childbirth preparation classes often use psychoprophylactic methods to reduce pain.
2. Teach the unprepared patient breathing techniques during early labor.
Rationale: Patients are more receptive to teaching during early labor.
3. Encourage the support person in methods that may help to reduce patient discomfort.
Rationale: Studies have shown that a support person helps to reduce the length of labor.
4. Provide comfort measures.
Rationale: Backrubs, massage, and other comfort measures help to reduce the discomfort of labor.
5. Administer an analgesic, as ordered.
Rationale: Medications are sometimes necessary to facilitate the physical and emotional progress of labor.
6. Assist in the placement of an epidural catheter, if ordered.
Rationale: Regional anesthesia provides analgesia and anesthesia during labor and delivery.

Nursing diagnosis

Fluid Volume Deficit related to insufficient intake during labor.
Desired outcome: Patient will maintain adequate hydration during labor.

Nursing interventions and rationales

1. Assess the patient's skin turgor, mucous membranes, and urine concentration.

Rationale: This assessment gives an indication of the degree of dehydration.

2. Administer fluids by mouth (if ordered and if tolerated by the patient) or I.V., as ordered.

Rationale: Administering fluids replaces lost fluids and maintains a state of hydration. Adequate hydration facilitates the normal labor process.

3. Monitor the patient's intake and output.

Rationale: Intake and output are indications of fluid balance in the body.

Nursing diagnosis

Decreased Cardiac Output related to maternal position during labor or epidural anesthesia

Desired outcome: Patient will maintain normal blood pressure and normal fetal heart-rate pattern during labor.

Nursing interventions and rationales

1. Encourage the patient to avoid the supine position.

Rationale: The uterus' pressure on the vena cava decreases blood flow into the right side of the heart, thus decreasing cardiac output and tissue perfusion. Side-lying position improves cardiac output.

2. Reload patients receiving epidural anesthesia with I.V. fluids (500-1,000 ml, as ordered).

Rationale: The increased intravascular volume will offset the drop in blood pressure produced by the epidural anesthesia.

3. Monitor the patient's blood pressure and pulse rate.

Rationale: Decreased blood pressure and increased pulse rate occur with vena cava syndrome; the patient should be monitored closely. Patients receiving an epidural block should have their blood pressure taken at least every 15 minutes.

4. Observe for changes in fetal heart rate and monitor pattern.

Rationale: Decreased placental perfusion decreases oxygen to the fetus, causing changes in the fetal heart rate.

Nursing diagnosis

Altered Nutrition: Less Than Body Requirements related to restricted intake during labor

Desired outcome: Patient will not develop ketosis during labor.

Nursing interventions and rationales

1. Provide fluids by mouth or I.V. (as ordered) during labor.

Rationale: Administering fluids provides a limited amount of glucose for energy.

2. Check the patient's urine for ketones.

Rationale: Ketones in the urine indicate maternal fat consumption for energy.

Nursing diagnosis

Altered Urinary Elimination related to pressure of the presenting part or to epidural anesthesia
Desired outcome: Patient will experience no significant bladder distention during labor.

Nursing interventions and rationales

1. Encourage voiding every 2 to 3 hours; assess for bladder distention frequently.
Rationale: The patient may be unaware of the need to void.
2. Monitor the patient's intake and output.
Rationale: Intake and output are indications of fluid balance.
3. Catheterize the patient, as ordered, if necessary.
Rationale: Patients are often unable to void during labor.

Nursing diagnosis

Ineffective Family Coping: compromised related to the labor process
Desired Outcome: Patient maintains control during labor.

Nursing interventions and rationales

1. Explain the equipment you are using and the procedures you are following, and keep the patient and her family updated on the process and progress of her labor.
Rationale: Keeping the patient and her family informed lessens anxiety.
2. Reinforce or suggest coping behaviors.
Rationale: The nurse is often able to identify behaviors that appear to have a positive effect on labor progress.
3. Provide support and encouragement for the support person (labor coach).
Rationale: The support person needs to feel that he or she is an essential part of the labor process.
4. Allow the patient to choose her own means of conducting the labor process (such as walking or showering) when possible.
Rationale: Allowing the patient choices enables her to maintain some degree of control over the labor process.

Nursing diagnosis

Knowledge Deficit related to the process of labor and birth
Desired outcome: Patient will obtain the information necessary to minimize the fear and anxieties associated with labor and to participate in the birth experience to the degree desired.

Nursing interventions and rationales

1. Orient the patient and her support person to the hospital environment.
Rationale: Unfamiliar surroundings can be a source of anxiety for the patient or her support person.

2. Explain all procedures and equipment, allowing the patient and support person to ask questions.
Rationale: Knowing what to expect helps lessen the anxiety.
3. Individualize teaching to the needs of the patient.
Rationale: Individualized teaching allows the nurse to concentrate on the specific needs of the patient.

☐ Assessment of the postpartum patient

The postpartum period, a time of major physiologic change, is the interval that occurs immediately after delivery until the time the reproductive organs have returned to a nonpregnant state. By recognizing the physiologic changes, which affect nearly every body system, you'll be able to deal effectively with the complications that may threaten the well-being of the mother or her newborn.

Immediate postpartum assessment

In most childbearing settings, the patient remains in the labor and delivery area after delivery for 1 to 2 hours of intense observation. At this time, the assessment focuses primarily on physiologic processes; however, it also provides the nurse with an opportunity to observe the early interactions between parents and their newborn.

The patient should be checked every 15 minutes for the first hour, then less frequently until transferred to the postpartum unit. However, patients who have experienced complications in labor or delivery or who are not progressing normally may require a longer period of intense observation.

The following information is important, especially if the postpartum nurse did not assist the patient during labor and delivery.

Gravida or para

Knowing the details about any poor outcomes the patient may have had with previous pregnancies is essential for the postpartum nurse to give specialized care. Patients who have had several previous deliveries are at increased risk for postpartum hemorrhage. First-time mothers may need special assistance and instruction.

Significant complications during pregnancy, labor, or delivery

Many complications require specialized care during the postpartum period. For example, anemic patients are at increased risk for infections and hemorrhage. Blood pressure elevations during labor require close monitoring in the postpartum period. A difficult delivery predisposes the patient to lacerations and hematoma formations.

Length of labor

A precipitate labor predisposes the patient to lacerations and uterine atony, whereas a long labor predisposes the patient to uterine atony, dehydration, and maternal exhaustion.

Induction and augmentation of labor
Use of oxytocin to stimulate labor predisposes the patient to postpartum hemorrhage.

Type of delivery
Patients who delivered by cesarean section will have an abdominal incision and may have less vaginal bleeding than those who delivered vaginally.

Birth weight
Large babies overdistend the uterus and predispose the patient to postpartum hemorrhage.

Analgesia and anesthesia
Patients who have had epidural anesthesia will be unable to walk until sensation to the legs returns; they are also more likely to have difficulties with voiding. General anesthesia may produce relaxation of the uterus and predispose the patient to postpartum hemorrhage.

Blood type and Rh factor
Rh-negative patients must be evaluated for the need for the administration of Rh immune globulin within 72 hours after delivery.

Rubella titer
Patients not immune to rubella should be immunized during the postpartum period.

Status of the newborn
If the newborn cannot room with the mother, the postpartum nurse must communicate actively with the nursery staff to keep abreast of any changes in the newborn's status.

Feeding preference
Breast-fed babies should be allowed to nurse early and often to establish good breast-feeding patterns, to help excrete bilirubin through meconium, and to decrease the amount of engorgement.

Physical assessment

If you're assisting the postpartum nurse, you may need to perform the physical assessment, which includes noting the following:

Vital signs
When taking the patient's blood pressure, note that:
• the patient's blood pressure should not change significantly during the postpartum period.
• hypotension indicates possible hypovolemia.
• the first signs of PIH may become apparent during the postpartum period.
    When taking the patient's temperature, keep in mind that:
• elevations up to 100.4° F (38° C) during the first 24 hours after

INVOLUTION OF THE UTERUS

For most postpartum patients, involution of the uterus occurs at a rate of about 1 cm/day after delivery.

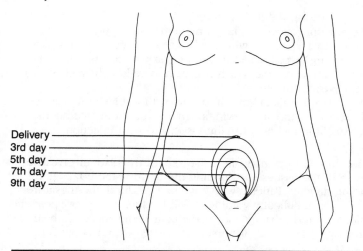

Delivery
3rd day
5th day
7th day
9th day

delivery may result from dehydration or a normal inflammatory response.
• elevations after the first 24 hours suggest sepsis, endometritis, urinary tract infection, mastitis, or another infection. An elevated temperature during this period should be reported to the health care provider for further evaluation.

When measuring the patient's pulse rate, note that:
• bradycardia is common for 6 to 8 days after delivery; a rate of 50 to 70 beats/minute is considered normal.
• pulse rates greater than normal may indicate infection or hypovolemia.

Respiratory rate should be within the normal range.

Fundus
The fundus should be at the level of the umbilicus after delivery and should descend approximately 1 cm/day thereafter (see *Involution of the uterus*). However, patients who breast-feed may experience a more rapid involution of the uterus as a result of the release of oxytocin from the posterior pituitary during nursing.

Keep the following points in mind when assessing the fundus:
• An elevated fundus that is displaced to the right suggests a full bladder.
• A flaccid fundus indicates uterine atony and should be massaged until firm.
• A tender fundus suggests an infection.

Many postpartum patients receive oxytocin in their I.V. fluids to prevent uterine atony. Review the postpartum order sheet for

any additional medications you'll need to administer to help minimize bleeding and promote involution of the uterus.

Lochia
When assessing the lochia, note:
• the amount (excessive, large, moderate, or scant)
• the character (rubra, which is bright red, occurs 1 to 3 days
postpartum; serosa, which is pink to brown, occurs 5 to 7 days
postpartum; and alba, which is cream to yellowish, occurs 1 to 3
weeks postpartum).

   Excessive lochia rubra that occurs with a relaxed uterus results from uterine atony; with a firm uterus, from lacerations.
Foul-smelling lochia is usually associated with infection.

Bladder
Labor and delivery may affect the tone of the bladder or cause
edema of the tissues surrounding the urethra, thereby making
voiding difficult. Patients who have had epidural anesthesia frequently have difficulty voiding. A full bladder may predispose the
patient to uterine atony and subsequent hemorrhage. Catheterization may be necessary if nursing measures are unsuccessful.

Perineum
Assess the perineum and episiotomy for redness, edema, ecchymoses, discharge, approximation of the wound edges, and pain.
Then, examine the anal area for hemorrhoids. If ordered, apply
ice packs to the perineum immediately after delivery to minimize edema and promote comfort. After the patient voids, provide warm sitz baths and heat, as ordered; this should provide
comfort, help minimize infection, and promote healing.

   After labor, the patient may experience a shaking chill, possibly caused by the sudden release of intra-abdominal pressure
that results from the emptying of the uterus at delivery. Warm
blankets and warm beverages may help to alleviate this common
occurrence.

Ongoing postpartum assessment
During the ongoing assessment, continue monitoring immediate
physical assessment areas and observe the following:

Breasts
For breast-feeding patients, note the following:
• Expect the patient to secrete colostrum for the first few days
after delivery. Then, on the 2nd or 3rd day postpartum, the
breasts should become tense as a result of the beginning of milk
production. Engorgement may occur on the 3rd or 4th day.
• Examine the breasts every 8 hours for signs of mastitis (heat,
pain, redness, or masses).
• Examine the nipples for shape, cracks, fissures, or soreness.
• Advise the patient to wear a well-fitting support bra 24 hours a
day.

ELICITING HOMANS' SIGN

To elicit this sign, first support the patient's thigh with one hand and her foot with the other. Bend her leg slightly at the knee, then firmly and abruptly dorsiflex the ankle. Resulting deep calf pain indicates a positive Homans' sign. (The patient may also resist ankle dorsiflexion or flex the knee involuntarily if Homans' sign is positive.)

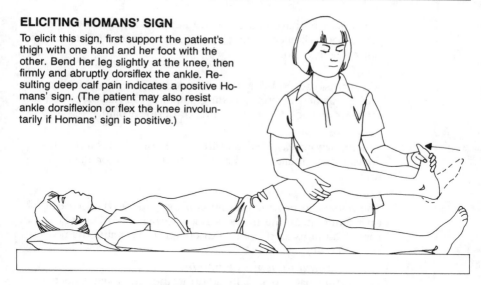

For bottle-feeding patients, note the following:
• Administer bromocriptine (Parlodel), as ordered, to suppress lactation.
• Examine the breasts for signs of engorgement, mastitis, or masses.

Extremities

Examine the patient's legs for edema, redness, heat, or a positive Homans' sign (see *Eliciting Homans' sign*). Because blood-clotting factors are increased during pregnancy, the patient may be predisposed to thromboembolism. Early ambulation promotes circulation to the extremities and helps minimize the incidence of thrombophlebitis.

Urine output

Marked diuresis begins within 12 hours after delivery. Check the bladder for distention every 4 to 6 hours; a full bladder may prevent uterine contraction and may predispose the patient to hemorrhage. Anesthesia or trauma during labor and delivery may predispose the patient to urine retention.

Elimination

Stool softeners, laxatives, suppositories, or enemas may be necessary for the postpartum patient. The patient may also benefit from a high-fiber diet to help stimulate peristalsis. Note the following:
• Decreased muscle tone during pregnancy may have predisposed the patient to constipation.
• Hemorrhoids, common during pregnancy, may have become aggravated by pushing in labor. Preventing constipation is essential for patients with hemorrhoids.

• Patients who have had extensive perineal repair should be given stool softeners daily to prevent trauma to the suture lines during defecation.

Pain
Afterpains, caused by uterine contractions, are most common in multiparas and in breast-feeding patients. You may need to administer analgesics for afterpains or perineal pain.

Nutrition
Patients who breast-feed require 500 extra calories a day, increased fluid intake, and should continue taking prenatal vitamins.

Contraception planning
The nurse can provide education if the patient has not decided on a family planning method. Both Norplant and Depo-Provera can be administered prior to discharge if the patient is not breast-feeding.

Emotional adjustment to parenting
Postpartum patients usually adjust to the emotional aspects of parenting in phases.

• During the first 2 days of the postpartum period (taking-in phase), the patient is frequently preoccupied with her own needs.
• Throughout the next 10 days (taking-hold phase), the patient strives for independence and is concerned about the return of normal bodily functions. Her first mothering tasks are important, and nursing support and encouragement are essential.
• Eventually, the patient realizes and accepts her physical separation from the baby and relinquishes her former role as a childless person (letting-go phase).

Evaluate the patient for signs of abnormal behavior, including persistent insomnia, lack of appetite, distant and aloof attitude toward her newborn, and excessive somatic complaints having no physical basis.

Laboratory data

Note the following information regarding test results for the postpartum patient:
• In many cases the patient's hematocrit level is falsely elevated because of a rapid loss of plasma.
• The white blood count usually increases during the postpartum period.
• Coagulation factors usually increase during pregnancy and the early postpartum period; this predisposes the patient to thrombophlebitis.
• Rh-negative patients must be evaluated for the need for Rh immune globulin. If the newborn is Rh-positive and the infant's direct Coombs' test is negative, $Rh_o(D)$ immune globulin must be given within 72 hours of delivery.

• If the patient is not immune to the rubella virus, vaccination should occur before discharge.

☐ Nursing diagnoses and interventions (postpartum)

Below is a list of the nursing diagnoses and interventions associated with the normal postpartum period.

Nursing diagnosis

High Risk for Infection of the Uterus or the Perineum related to trauma or surgical incision
Desired outcome: Patient will not develop an infection during the postpartum period.

Nursing interventions and rationales

1. Monitor the patient's temperature and pulse rate frequently.
Rationale: Increased temperature and pulse rate are signs of infection. However, the patient's temperature may be as high as 100.4° F (38° C) during the first 24 hours after delivery as a result of dehydration or inflammation.
2. Observe the perineal area for redness, edema, discharge, or pain.
Rationale: These may be signs of perineal infection.
3. Monitor the fundus for tenderness and the lochia for odor.
Rationale: These may be signs of uterine infection.
4. Perform perineal care, as ordered.
Rationale: Regular cleansing of the perineal area removes bacteria; heat increases circulation to the area, which promotes healing.
5. Apply perineal pads from the front to the back; remove them in the same manner.
Rationale: This method avoids contaminating the perineal area with bacteria from the rectum.
6. Take the proper measures to minimize exposing the patient to infection from the hospital staff (for example, by washing hands and changing into scrub gown).
Rationale: The hospital staff can be a source of infection for the patient.

Nursing diagnosis

High Risk for Infection of the Breast related to milk stasis
Desired outcome: Patient will not develop mastitis.

Nursing interventions and rationales

1. If the patient has elected to breast-feed the newborn, encourage her to nurse frequently.
Rationale: Frequent emptying of the breasts prevents milk stasis, an excellent medium for bacterial growth.

2. Examine the patient's nipples every 8 hours for cracks or abrasions.
Rationale: Breaks in the skin provide an entry for bacteria.
3. Examine the patient's breasts every 8 hours for signs of mastitis (redness, heat, pain).
Rationale: Early intervention can prevent further complications, such as abscess formation.
4. To help prevent engorgement, encourage frequent breast-feeding or manual expression of milk. If the patient is bottle-feeding, administer lactation suppressants, as ordered.
Rationale: Stasis of milk in the breast provides an excellent medium for bacterial growth.
5. Advise the patient to change nursing positions periodically (for example, lying, sitting, then a football-carry position).
Rationale: Changing position ensures thorough emptying of all milk ducts.

Nursing diagnosis
Fluid Volume Deficit related to hemorrhage
Desired outcome: Patient will experience no significant blood loss in the postpartum period.

Nursing interventions and rationales
1. Monitor the fundus for position and consistency.
Rationale: If uterine atony occurs, prompt massage will prevent excessive blood loss.
2. Monitor the amount and consistency of lochia.
Rationale: An excessive amount with frequent large clots requires intervention to prevent further blood loss.
3. Monitor the patient's blood pressure and pulse rate.
Rationale: Decreased blood pressure and increased pulse rate suggest hypovolemia.
4. Monitor the patient's bladder function and take measures to prevent distention.
Rationale: A full bladder prevents adequate uterine contraction.
5. Administer oxytocic medications, as ordered.
Rationale: Such medications help keep the uterus contracted.

Nursing diagnosis
Pain related to episiotomy, afterpains, or hemorrhoids
Desired outcome: Nursing measures and/or medication will provide the patient with relief from discomfort.

Nursing interventions and rationales
1. Assess the location, severity, and duration of the patient's pain.
Rationale: Excessive perineal or vaginal pain may indicate hematoma formation, lacerations, or infection.

2. Provide comfort measures, such as a sitz bath, local anesthetics, and pain medication, as ordered.
Rationale: Pain may affect the mother's ability to interact with her newborn.
3. Help the patient prevent constipation.
Rationale: Hard stool will be painful if the patient has an episiotomy or hemorrhoids.

Nursing diagnosis
Altered Urinary Elimination related to childbirth
Desired outcome: Patient will maintain normal bladder function during the postpartum period.

Nursing interventions and rationales
1. Ambulate the patient to the bathroom to void as soon as possible after delivery.
Rationale: Patients usually find it easier to void on the commode.
2. Apply ice to the perineum during the first 24 hours, then heat as ordered.
Rationale: Minimizing edema will prevent urine retention caused by obstruction.
3. Monitor the position of the fundus.
Rationale: A fundus that is raised and displaced to the right suggests a full bladder.

Nursing diagnosis
Constipation related to pregnancy changes, medications, and perineal trauma
Desired outcome: Patient will reestablish a normal bowel pattern prior to discharge.

Nursing interventions and rationales
1. Administer stool softeners or laxatives, as ordered.
Rationale: Patients often need medication to help keep stools soft and to stimulate peristalsis.
2. Encourage a high-fiber diet.
Rationale: Fiber provides bulk in the intestine and promotes normal bowel function.
3. Encourage the patient to consume fluids.
Rationale: Inadequate fluid intake predisposes the patient to harder stool formation.
4. Encourage the patient to walk.
Rationale: Walking stimulates intestinal peristalsis.

Nursing diagnosis
Knowledge Deficit related to conception, parenthood, postpartum changes, or infant care

Desired outcome: Patient will obtain the knowledge she needs to care for herself and her infant as well as to make a satisfying emotional and physical adjustment during the postpartum period.

Nursing interventions and rationales
1. Assess the patient's educational needs.
Rationale: This will help you to identify the appropriate focus for postpartum teaching.
2. Provide classes, demonstrations, or reading materials to meet the patient's needs.
Rationale: People learn by a variety of educational strategies.
3. Follow up the teaching session with return demonstrations and question-and-answer sessions to assess the level of knowledge obtained.
Rationale: Follow-up sessions will help in evaluating the educational strategies and in planning further instruction.

☐ Assessment and care of the newborn
During the first few days of extrauterine life, the newborn undergoes profound physiologic changes. Although most newborns adapt readily to the environment, you'll need to perform frequent assessments to determine how well he is managing.

Risk assessment
Performed by the nurse who plans to care for the newborn after delivery, risk assessment works on the principle that most risk factors affecting the mother will also affect the newborn. By using this information, the nurse can anticipate potential problems, thereby allowing her sufficient time to prepare for possible complications. However, if the nurse anticipates the newborn to be severely depressed or expects to find meconium-stained fluid, additional specialized help will be needed in the delivery room.
    When performing a risk assessment, note the following:
Mother's age
Teenagers are at risk for delivering low-birth-weight infants. Patients over age 35 are at increased risk for having children with chromosomal abnormalities.
Family history
Certain diseases and anomalies may be inherited.
Previous obstetric history
The newborn should be assessed for problems that may have occurred during the patient's previous pregnancies.
Prenatal care
Lack of prenatal care places the patient and her newborn at risk.
Weight gain
Poor or excessive weight gain may lead to neonatal problems,

including growth retardation or macrosomia. The nurse should be alerted to the possibility of shoulder dystocia if maternal weight gain has been excessive.

Maternal medication use and substance abuse
Medications taken during pregnancy, such as anticonvulsants, can cause anomalies in the infant. Newborns of substance-abusing patients should be monitored for signs of withdrawal.

Maternal prenatal and intrapartum complications
Such disorders potentiate fetal or neonatal complications.

Results of prenatal testing
Maternal laboratory studies and any fetal surveillance testing should be noted as well as maternal blood type and Rh factor.

Length of gestation
Pre- and post-term newborns are at increased risk for complications.

Length and character of labor
Precipitate or prolonged labor should be noted.

Length of membrane rupture
Prolonged rupture of the membranes places the newborn at risk for infection.

Amount of amniotic fluid
Decreased amounts are associated with postmature infants and abnormalities of the urinary tract; increased amounts, with abnormalities of the upper GI tract.

Analgesia and anesthesia
Analgesics given close to the time of delivery may depress fetal respiratory centers. General anesthetics may depress the newborn; regional anesthetics may cause maternal hypotension and fetal distress.

Factors indicating possible fetal distress
Such factors include fetal monitoring patterns, scalp pH (if performed), and meconium in amniotic fluid (see *Normal umbilical cord blood gas values*, page 44, and "Scalp pH [fetal]" in Section 3).

Type of delivery
Newborns delivered by cesarean section are at increased risk for respiratory distress from fluid retained in the lungs. Those delivered by forceps are at increased risk for injuries. Those delivered by vacuum extraction are predisposed to cephalohematoma.

Delivery room assessment and care
Immediately after birth, while the newborn is still in the delivery room, the following assessment data should be obtained:

Apgar score
Performed 1 minute, then 5 minutes after birth, the Apgar score

NORMAL UMBILICAL CORD BLOOD GAS VALUES

Value	Artery	Vein
pH	7.24 ± 0.07	7.32 ± 0.06
PO_2 (mm Hg)	17.9 ± 6.9	28.7 ± 7.3
PCO_2 (mm Hg)	56.3 ± 8.6	43.8 ± 6.7
Bicarbonate (mEq/liter)	24.1 ± 2.2	22.6 ± 2.1
Base excess (mEq/liter)	−3.6 ± 2.7	−2.9 ± 2.4

enables quick evaluation of the newborn's condition. A score of 7 to 10 indicates the newborn is in good condition; 4 to 6, fair condition; and 0 to 3, extremely poor condition (see *Understanding the Apgar scoring system*).

Post-delivery nursing measures

The following measures should be performed in the delivery room:
• Establish and maintain a patent airway. Be sure to:
  — suction the newborn's mouth, then nares with a bulb syringe
  — dry the newborn and stimulate crying by rubbing him.
  — maintain a modified Trendelenburg position to facilitate drainage of mucus.
• Prevent hypothermia. To do so:
  — dry the newborn thoroughly
  — place him under a radiant warmer
  — place a stockinette cap on the newborn's head.
• Identify the newborn.
• Promote early maternal-newborn attachment.

General physical data

For this brief assessment, be sure to note the following data:
• Observe for obvious defects or evidence of trauma.
• Check the skin for color, staining, or peeling.
• Note whether the cord has three vessels.
• Check the nostrils for patency.
• Auscultate the heart and lungs.
• Palpate the liver for enlargement and the chest for point of maximum cardiac impulse.

Neonatal care in the transitional period

The transitional period—the first 6 to 8 hours after delivery—can be extremely hazardous to the newborn. During this time, the newborn is usually transferred from the delivery room to a spe-

UNDERSTANDING THE APGAR SCORING SYSTEM

To quickly evaluate a newborn's condition, use the Apgar scoring system shown in the chart below. This reliable, widely accepted scoring system allows you to readily establish a baseline evaluation.

Quickly assess the newborn 1 minute after birth and again 5 minutes later. During each assessment, evaluate the five vital indicators (heart rate, respiratory effort, muscle tone, reflex irritability, and skin color), rating each 0 (very poor) to 2 (excellent). Add the points to determine the infant's total score. A score of 7 to 10 indicates excellent condition; 4 to 6, fair condition; and 0 to 3, very poor condition. An infant who scores less than 6 may require immediate resuscitation.

Note the following:
• *Heart rate.* This indicator is the most important—and the last to be absent if a newborn is in distress. Within the first few minutes after birth, normal heart rate is 150 to 180 beats/minute. It then subsides to 130 to 140 beats/minute. (Such activities as crying

temporarily raise heart rate). Consider a heart rate below 100 beats/minute to indicate asphyxia. Closely observe the newborn and prepare to resuscitate him, if needed.

For the most accurate assessment, determine apical heart rate with a pediatric stethoscope.
• *Respiratory effort.* Within 1 or 2 minutes after birth, the newborn should breathe spontaneously and regularly, at a rate of 30 to 60 breaths/minute (bpm).
• *Muscle tone.* Expect a newborn with good muscle tone to maintain constant flexion of his arms and legs and to resist your efforts to straighten them.
• *Reflex irritability.* A newborn should protest during suctioning—the louder, the better. You may also test reflex irritabiliy by gently tapping his foot and noting how vigorously he responds.
• *Skin color.* All newborns are cyanotic at birth, but a normal infant's body becomes pink (if he's Caucasian or Asian) within 3 minutes. His extremities, however, may remain blue for a while longer.

Indicator	0	1	2
Heart rate	Absent	Less than 100 bpm	More than 100 bpm
Respiratory effort	Absent	Slow, irregular, weak cry	Good, vigorous cry
Muscle tone	Flaccid, limp	Some flexion of extremities	Good flexion, active motion
Reflex irritability (in response to catheter in nostril)	No response	Weak cry or grimace	Vigorous cry, cough, sneeze
Skin color	Blue	Body skin normal (depending on the newborn's race), extremities blue	Body and extremity skin color normal

cialized area where he is monitored closely (if staffing and facilities permit, the newborn can be monitored in the patient's room). After he has been thoroughly examined, assessed for gestational age, and given any necessary medications, the newborn can be returned to the patient's room as long as his condition is stable.

Physical examination

Assessment during the transitional period should include the following:

Vital signs

When monitoring the newborn's temperature, keep in mind the following information:

• Some facilities recommend taking an initial rectal temperature to assure anal patency. (Normal rectal temperature is 97.8° to 99° F [36.5° to 37.2°C]).

• Axillary temperature should be 97.6° to 98.6° F (36.4° to 37° C).

• The newborn should be kept under a radiant warmer to conserve heat.

• The newborn should not be bathed until his temperature has stabilized.

When assessing the apical pulse, note that a rate of 100 beats/minute when the newborn is sleeping and 180 beats/minute when crying is considered normal (the range is usually 120 to 160 beats/minute). Be sure to auscultate for murmurs and arrhythmias.

When assessing respirations, keep in mind that a rate of 30 to 60 respirations/minute is normal and that the rate is normally irregular. Auscultate the newborn's lungs for crackles, rhonchi, wheezing, and grunting. Also, observe for nasal flaring or retractions, both signs of respiratory distress.

Body measurements

For a term newborn, the following measurements are considered normal:

• weight: 7 to 8 lb (3.2 to 3.6 kg)

• length: approximately 18″ to 22″ (45.7 to 55.9 cm)

• head circumference: 12½″ to 14½″ (31.8 to 36.8 cm). A head circumference of less than 12½″ (32 cm) may indicate premature birth or microcephaly; a circumference that is more than 1½″ (3.8 cm) larger than that of the chest may indicate hydrocephaly.

• chest circumference: 12″ to 13″ (30.5 to 33 cm). Chest circumference is usually about ¾″ (1.9 cm) less than that of the head.

Skin

When assessing skin color, note the following:

• Acrocyanosis (cyanotic discoloration of the extremities) is a common result of poor peripheral circulation.

• A dark red color is common in premature infants.

• Pallor may indicate central nervous system damage, cardiovascular problems, blood dyscrasia, blood loss, or infection.

• Cyanosis is common in newborns with hypothermia, infection, hypoglycemia, cardiopulmonary diseases, and cardiac, neurologic, or respiratory malformations.

• Petechiae over the presenting part result from pressure. Petechiae over other areas may indicate infection or clotting-factor deficiency.

• Ecchymoses may be caused by forceps in vertex presentations; those occurring in breech presentations usually appear on the legs and buttocks.

• Jaundice normally occurs 36 to 72 hours after delivery. Jaundice occurring before this time may indicate early hemolysis of red blood cells and must be reported.

When assessing birthmarks, keep in mind the following information:
• Mongolian spots are normally present in 70% of Black, Asian, and Native American newborns and in 9% of White newborns.
• The location and size of hemangiomas should be noted.
• Café-au-lait spots may indicate neurofibromatosis.

When assessing skin condition, note that premature infants frequently have thin skin with many blood vessels as a result of a lack of subcutaneous fat, whereas postmature newborns frequently have thick skin that is parchmentlike, peeling, and often meconium-stained.

Lanugo and vernix are usually absent in postmature newborns; abundant or excessive in premature newborns.

Head

The anterior fontanelle usually closes by the time the infant is 18 months old. Bulging indicates possible increased intracranial pressure; depression indicates dehydration. The posterior fontanel may be closed at birth.

Conditions affecting the newborn's head include the following:
• hydrocephalus, in which sutures are widely spaced because of dilation of the cerebral ventricles
• synostosis (premature closure of the sutures), which requires medical intervention
• caput succedaneum, a benign condition characterized by soft-tissue edema from pressure during labor that crosses the suture lines of the skull
• cephalohematoma, resulting from an accumulation of blood between the bone and periosteum usually appearing within the first 2 days; it does not cross suture lines. Expect increased bilirubin level and jaundice as the condition resolves.

Eyes

Widely spaced or closely set eyes are associated with some genetic disorders. Several chromosomal diseases have characteristic abnormalities of the eyes. Opacity of the lens or absence of the red reflex may indicate congenital cataracts. Discharge from the eye may indicate chlamydial or gonorrheal conjunctivitis.

Nose

Choanal atresia, a congenital blockage in the posterior nares, prohibits normal exchange of air because newborns are obligate nose-breathers. Drainage or malformation of the nose is associated with congenital syphilis.

Mouth

When assessing the newborn's mouth, check the hard and soft palates for clefts. Also check for teeth and for the gag reflex before the initial feeding. Note that excessive saliva may be from esophageal atresia or tracheoesophageal fistula. White plaques may be caused by thrush (candidal infection).

Ears

Check for patency of the ear canals. Note that low-set ears are associated with trisomy 21 (Down syndrome). The presence of skin tags is sometimes associated with other anomalies.

Neck

Webbing is associated with Turner's syndrome.

Chest

When assessing the chest, note whether the newborn has gynecomastia, caused by maternal hormones, or supernumerary nipples. Also, palpate the clavicles for fractures. Note that breath and heart sounds are assessed along with other vital signs.

Abdomen

Keep in mind that the newborn's umbilical cord should be clamped for at least the first 24 hours after birth. Expect the cord to have two arteries and one vein. The presence of only one artery is frequently associated with other abnormalities, especially of the genitourinary tract, and should be reported to the health care provider at once.

Other cord abnormalities may include:
- a bleeding cord, which may indicate hemorrhagic disease
- redness or drainage, which may indicate infection
- an umbilical hernia
- meconium staining, which indicates passage of meconium before labor
- a small, thin cord, which may be associated with poor fetal growth.

When assessing the abdomen further, note any distention (obstruction, mass, or sepsis) or depression (diaphragmatic hernia). Be sure to palpate the femoral pulse: a weak or absent femoral pulse may indicate hip dysplasia or coarctation of the aorta. Expect to hear bowel sounds within 1 or 2 hours after birth.

Genitals

If the newborn is female, blood-tinged discharge may be present from the vagina as a result of maternal hormone withdrawal. Note the first voiding, which should occur within the first 24 hours.

If the newborn is male, note the position of the urinary meatus: hypospadias refers to the opening appearing on the bottom of the penis; epispadias refers to the opening appearing on top of the penis. Palpate the scrotum for the presence of testes; in many premature newborns, the testes will not have descended. Note the first voiding, which should occur within the first 24 hours.

Anus

Check the newborn's anus for patency. Note the first stool (meconium), which should pass within the first 24 hours.

Extremities
Note the following information:
• Poor muscle tone is associated with prematurity or with the effect of maternally administered drugs during labor.
• Lack of movement or asymmetrical movement may indicate fracture, nerve trauma, or malformations.
• Extra or missing digits, as well as webbed digits, are associated with several anomalies.
• Simian creases are associated with trisomy 21 (Down syndrome).
• Occasional, slight tremors are common but may be a sign of hypoglycemia or drug withdrawal. Prolonged tremors may indicate central nervous system disorder.
• Major gluteal folds should be even. When thighs are rotated outward, no click should be felt. Abnormalities may indicate hip dysplasia.
• Acrocyanosis of feet and hands is common.

Back
The newborn's spine should be straight and easily flexed. If born at term, he should be able to raise and support his head momentarily when prone. Note pigmented nevi, hair tufts, and coccygeal dimples over the spine; they are often associated with spina bifida occulta.

Reflexes
Assessment of the newborn's reflexes provides useful information regarding the nervous system and the state of neurologic maturation. Reflexes such as sucking and swallowing are necessary for survival. Some other reflexes the nurse may observe are the rooting, grasp, and Moro reflex.

Gestational age assessment
Performed during the transitional period, gestational age assessment includes an examination of physical characteristics and neuromuscular development that should be done during the first 24 hours after birth; data collected before or after that may be insufficient for an accurate estimation of gestational age. (See *Ballard gestational-age assessment tool,* page 50.)

Medication administration
During the newborn period, administer the following prophylactic medications:

Neonatal eye prophylaxis
A prophylactic agent against *Chlamydia* and gonorrhea should be placed in the infant's eyes within 1 hour after birth. *Note:* Silver nitrate is ineffective against *Chlamydia.*

Prophylaxis of hemorrhagic disease in the newborn
Vitamin K is administered to all normal newborns to assist with blood clotting during the first week of life.

BALLARD GESTATIONAL-AGE ASSESSMENT TOOL

	-1	0	1	2	3	4	5

NEUROMUSCULAR MATURITY

	-1	0	1	2	3	4	5
Posture	—						—
Square window (wrist)	>90°	90°	60°	45°	30°	0°	—
Arm recoil	—	180°	140° to 180°	110° to 140°	90° to 110°	<90°	—
Popliteal angle	180°	160°	140°	120°	100°	90°	<90°
Scarf sign							
Heel to ear							—

PHYSICAL MATURITY

	-1	0	1	2	3	4	5
Skin	Sticky, friable, transparent	Gelatinous, red, trans-lucent	Smooth, pink; visible vessels	Superficial peeling or rash; few vis-ible vessels	Cracking; pale areas; rare visible vessels	Parchment-like; deep cracking; no visible vessels	Leathery, cracked, wrinkled
Lanugo	None	Sparse	Abundant	Thinning	Bald areas	Mostly bald	—
Plantar surface	Heel-toe 40 to 50 mm: -1; <40 mm: -2	>50 mm; no crease	Faint red marks	Anterior transverse crease only	Creases over anterior two-thirds	Creases over entire sole	—
Breast	Imperceptible	Barely perceptible	Flat areola, no bud	Stippled areola; 1- to 2-mm bud	Raised areola; 3- to 4-mm bud	Full areola; 5- to 10-mm bud	—
Eye and ear	Lids fused loosely: -1; tightly: -2	Lids open; pinna flat, stays folded	Slightly curved pinna; soft, slow recoil	Well-curved pinna; soft but ready recoil	Formed and firm; instant recoil	Thick car-tilage; ear stiff	—
Genitalia, male	Scrotum flat, smooth	Scrotum empty; faint rugae	Testes in upper canal; rare rugae	Testes de-scending; few rugae	Testes down; good rugae	Testes pen-dulous; deep rugae	—
Genitalia, female	Clitoris prom-inent; labia flat	Prominent clitoris; small labia minora	Prominent clitoris; en-larging minora	Majora and minora equally prom-inent	Majora large; minora small	Majora cover clitoris and minora	

MATURITY RATING

Score	-10	-5	0	5	10	15	20	25	30	35	40	45	50
Weeks	20	22	24	26	28	30	32	34	36	38	40	42	44

SCORING SECTION   1st Exam=X   2nd Exam=0

Estimating gestational age by maturity rating	_____ Weeks	_____ Weeks
Time of exam	Date _____ Hour _____ a.m. p.m.	Date _____ Hour _____ a.m. p.m.
Age at exam	_____ Hours	_____ Hours
Signature of examiner	_____ M.D.	_____ M.D.

Gestation by dates _____ Weeks

Birth date _____ Hour _____ a.m. p.m.

APGAR _____ 1 min _____ 5 min

Adapted from Ballard, J.L., Khoury, J.C., Wedig, K., et al. (1991). "New Ballard Score, expanded to include extremely premature infants." *Journal of Pediatrics*, 119(3): 417-423. Used with permission from Mosby, Inc.

PERFORMING A HEEL-STICK TEST

When performing a heel-stick test, first improve the infant's surface blood flow by warming his foot in the palm of your hand or wrapping the foot in a warm, moist compress for 3 to 5 minutes. Then, cleanse the foot with alcohol and allow it to dry. Using a disposable lancet, make a quick, clean stick on the outer surface of the heel. Then, after wiping the area with a gauze pad, collect the droplets of blood on a test strip for blood glucose testing.

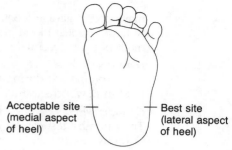

Acceptable site
(medial aspect
of heel)

Best site
(lateral aspect
of heel)

Hepatitis B vaccine
The CDC recommends hepatitis B vaccine to begin for newborns within 48 hours of birth. Infants born to chronic carriers also are given hepatitis B immune globulin within 12 hours of birth.

Laboratory tests

Certain tests may be performed routinely during the transitional period, including the following:

Blood glucose screening
Blood glucose screening may be performed on all newborns or only on those identified to be at risk for hypoglycemia. Those at risk include the following:
• newborns weighing more than 8 lb, 13 oz (4 kg) or less than 5 lb, 10 oz (2.6 kg)
• growth-retarded infants
• infants of diabetic or preeclamptic patients
• polycythemic, cold-stressed, or postmature infants
• infants with severe erythroblastosis fetalis or congenital heart disease
• infants of patients who received dextrose infusions during labor.

Signs and symptoms include feeding difficulty, hunger, cyanosis, apnea, lethargy, a weak, high-pitched cry, jitteriness, twitching, eye rolling, and convulsions.

To determine whether the infant is hypoglycemic, you'll need to perform a heel-stick test (see *Performing a heel-stick test*). If results indicate hypoglycemia, a venipuncture should be performed and sent to the laboratory to verify results. Values for hypoglycemia are as follows:
• less than 30 mg/dl during first 72 hours of life
• less than 45 mg/dl after the first 3 days
• less than 20 mg/dl in premature infants.

If the infant has a good sucking or swallowing reflex, the infant can be fed according to hospital policy (dextrose 10% in water is frequently given). However, if the infant cannot take fluids by mouth, shows signs of respiratory distress, or the glucose concentration is extremely low, the health care provider may order a gavage feeding of dextrose 10% or I.V. glucose. Note that repeat blood glucose testing should be done after treatment of hypoglycemia.

Hematocrit levels
Not a routine test during the transitional period, the hematocrit level in newborns averages about 55%.

Coombs' test
The Coombs' test can be either indirect or direct. The indirect Coombs' test measures circulating antibodies and is more typically done on the mother (most know it as an antibody screen). The direct Coombs' test reveals the presence of antibodies attached to the red blood cells (RBCs). This attachment of antibodies causes the RBCs to be destroyed, producing hyperbilirubinemia and anemia in the neonate.

The direct Coombs' test will be performed on the cord blood if the mother is Rh negative or if the mother's blood is known to contain other antibodies (such as Kell, Duffy or Kidd) that cause hemolysis of fetal RBCs. This test also can be performed on the neonate after delivery if jaundice develops early in life (first 24 hours) or if the jaundice becomes severe during the neonatal period.

Bilirubin
Infants who develop jaundice early in life (first 24 hours), those with severe jaundice during the neonatal period, and those born to women with known pathological antibodies will need to have their bilirubin levels taken periodically. (See "Hyperbilirubinemia" in Section 2.)

Newborn screening tests
Most states require newborns to be screened for certain defects. Newborn screening tests detect disorders that can cause mental retardation, physical handicaps, or death if left undiscovered and untreated. The disorders that can be identified from several drops of blood obtained by a heel stick include galactosemia, homocystinuria, hypothyroidism, maple syrup urine disease, phenylketonuria (PKU), and sickle cell anemia. Because adequate protein intake is required for evaluation for PKU, a second test may be required if the first specimen was taken prior to several days of adequate breast- or bottle-feeding.

Ongoing newborn assessment
The following assessments should be made at the beginning of each 8-hour shift as long as the infant is hospitalized:
• axillary temperature
• respiratory rate, rhythm, effort, and breath sounds
• heart rate and rhythm
• skin color and condition
• activity

- tone
- feeding pattern
- elimination
- weight (the average newborn loses 10% of birth weight within the first few days of life; newborns are normally weighed only once a day).

General nursing care

The following nursing measures should be taken as part of the ongoing newborn assessment:

Maintaining a clear airway

When suctioning the airway, place the newborn in a side-lying or prone position. Using a bulb syringe (keep one handy in the infant's crib), always suction the mouth first. Stimulation of the nares initiates a gasp response that can pull mucus from the mouth into the lower airway.

Preventing hypothermia

Make sure the room temperature is kept at 75° F (23.9° C). Keep the newborn dry and wrapped, making sure the head is covered; the head represents a large portion of the newborn's body surface area. When performing procedures that require undressing the newborn, be sure to do them under a radiant warmer.

Cord care

The umbilical clamp can usually be removed after 24 hours. Apply the prescribed preparations (triple blue dye, alcohol) to the cord according to hospital policy. Keep the diaper from covering the cord.

Skin care

When bathing the newborn, use mild soap. Common skin conditions include erythema toxicum or neonatorum, a normal rash occurring during the first 3 weeks of life; and milia neonatorum, clogged sebaceous glands on the face.

Circumcision

Before a newborn is circumcised, the parents must give their written consent. (See Section 3, "Circumcision.")

Physiologic jaundice

First noticeable in the newborn's head, then progressing toward the abdomen and extremities, physiologic jaundice occurs after the first 24 hours of life and peaks at about the fifth day. The bilirubin level rises as the jaundice progresses; levels should not exceed 12 mg/dl.

Keep in mind the following information when caring for a newborn with jaundice:

- Breast-fed infants often have higher bilirubin levels because of the delay in milk production after delivery, especially if their mothers have not been able to breast-feed immediately after delivery. Early feeding tends to keep the bilirubin level low by stimulating intestinal activity.

• Hypothermia tends to increase bilirubin levels.
• Maternal ingestion of salicylates and sulfa drugs during the third trimester causes increased bilirubin levels.
• Infants of diabetic mothers tend to have higher bilirubin levels.
• Kernicterus refers to brain damage caused by high bilirubin levels. (Levels greater than 20 mg/dl in newborns born at term are associated with the risk of neurologic impairment.)

Although treatment is usually not required for physiologic jaundice, phototherapy may be used if levels reach the upper limits of normal. Nursing guidelines for phototherapy include the following:
• Expose as much skin area as possible to light.
• Protect the infant's eyes with patches.
• Use a paper face mask with the metal nose strip removed as a diaper.
• Monitor the infant's skin temperature.
• Note the frequency and type of stools; expect loose, greenish stools.
• Increase the newborn's fluid volume by 25% to prevent dehydration.
• Allow or encourage the mother to feed the newborn to help foster the attachment process. (For more information, see "Hyperbilirubinemia" in Section 2 and "Phototherapy" in Section 3.)

☐ Nursing diagnoses and interventions (neonatal)

Here is a listing of the nursing diagnoses and interventions frequently associated with the normal newborn infant.

Nursing diagnosis

High Risk for Infection related to immature immune system
Desired outcome: Infant will not develop a nosocomial infection while hospitalized.

Nursing interventions and rationales

1. Wear appropriate attire when handling the newborn.
Rationale: By wearing the appropriate attire, you can avoid introducing infection from clothing worn outside the nursery.
2. Be sure to scrub before entering the nursery and to wash hands before touching another infant.
Rationale: Scrubbing reduces bacteria present on the skin. Washing hands helps prevent transmission of organisms from one infant to another.
3. Avoid the nursery area if you have signs or symptoms of a potentially communicable disorder.
Rationale: A nurse may be a source of infection to the infant.
4. Cleanse the newborn's umbilical cord, as ordered, and observe for signs of infection.

Rationale: The cord is a potential port of entry for infection.
5. Observe the newborn's circumcision for signs of infection.
Rationale: Surgical incision is a potential port of entry for infection.
6. Check the newborn's skin for signs of infection (rash, vesicles, lesions).
Rationale: A newborn's skin is sensitive and susceptible to invasion by organisms.
7. Apply eye prophylaxis according to hospital policy.
Rationale: Eye prophylaxis destroys organisms that cause neonatal conjunctivitis.

Nursing diagnosis
Ineffective Airway Clearance related to mucus secretions
Desired outcome: Infant will establish a normal respiratory pattern during the transitional period.

Nursing interventions and rationales
1. Maintain the newborn in modified Trendelenburg's position after delivery.
Rationale: This position facilitates drainage of secretions.
2. Suction the newborn with a bulb syringe, as necessary.
Rationale: Removal of mucus will prevent aspiration into deeper respiratory structures and clear the airway.
3. Maintain the newborn in a side-lying or prone position.
Rationale: These positions help to prevent aspiration of mucus.
4. Observe the newborn's respiratory rate; auscultate the lungs for abnormal breath sounds. Also observe for nasal flaring, grunting, and retractions.
Rationale: Recognition of abnormal respiratory signs and symptoms allows for early intervention and prevention of complications.

Nursing diagnosis
Hypothermia related to exposure after birth
Desired outcome: Infant will maintain an axillary temperature between 97.6° to 98.6° F (36.4° to 37° C) during the newborn period.

Nursing interventions and rationales
1. Dry the newborn thoroughly after the delivery.
Rationale: Drying the newborn thoroughly will reduce heat loss by evaporation.
2. Place the newborn under a radiant warmer or wrap him in a warm blanket.
Rationale: This protects the newborn from the coolness of the delivery room, which can cause rapid body cooling.
3. Cover the newborn's head with a cap.
Rationale: The head represents a large portion of the newborn's

body surface area; exposure of the head causes significant heat loss.

4. Avoid bathing the newborn when his temperature is low.
Rationale: Bathing further lowers temperature through the heat loss caused by evaporation and exposure.

5. Monitor the newborn's temperature frequently.
Rationale: Early recognition and correction of hypothermia can prevent further complications, such as hypoglycemia.

Nursing diagnosis

High Risk for Injury related to hyperbilirubinemia
Desired outcome: The newborn's bilirubin levels will not exceed 12 mg/dl.

Nursing interventions and rationales

1. Monitor the newborn's skin color and the progression of jaundice
Rationale: The degree and extent of jaundice are indications of bilirubin level.

2. Encourage early, regular feeding.
Rationale: Early feeding stimulates intestinal activity, which helps to eliminate bilirubin in the stool.

3. Take measures to prevent hypothermia.
Rationale: Hypothermia tends to increase bilirubin levels.

Nursing diagnosis

High Risk for Injury related to hypoglycemia
Desired outcome: Newborn will maintain a blood glucose level above 30 mg/dl during the first 72 hours.

Nursing interventions and rationales

1. Promote early, frequent feeding.
Rationale: Early feeding supplies glucose, which may prevent hypoglycemia.

2. Monitor the newborn for signs of hypoglycemia and obtain glucose levels, as ordered.
Rationale: Early intervention prevents complications.

3. Take measures to prevent hypothermia.
Rationale: Hypothermia increases glucose utilization in an attempt to maintain body temperature, thereby lowering blood glucose levels.

2 Complications and Disorders

In this section, you'll find an alphabetical listing of some of the most commonly encountered complications and disorders of pregnancy and the neonate along with related nursing diagnoses and interventions.

☐ Abruptio placentae

Abruptio placentae refers to the separation of a normally im-planted placenta from the uterine wall after the 20th week of gestation and before the fetus is delivered (see *Total abruptio placentae,* page 58). Bleeding may appear in the vagina or may be concealed behind the placenta. Shock, fetal distress or death, uteroplacental apoplexy (Couvelaire uterus), and disseminated intravascular coagulation (DIC) may occur. Maternal mortality is about 1%; fetal mortality may be as high as 25% to 50%.

Predisposing factors include the following:
• trauma
• short umbilical cord
• uterine anomaly
• maternal hypertension
• vena cava syndrome
• cigarette smoking
• previous abruptio placentae
• high parity
• maternal age over 30
• sudden uterine decompression
• polyhydramnios
• use of injectable drugs, specifically cocaine.

Frequently-encountered data for abruptio placentae include the following:

Subjective data
• abdominal pain and tenderness

Objective data
• vaginal bleeding
• boardlike rigidity of the abdomen
• abnormal or absent fetal heart tones
• hypotension
• tachycardia
• pallor
• cool, moist skin
• bloody amniotic fluid
• increased resting tone of the uterus
• rising fundal height from blood trapped behind the placenta

TOTAL ABRUPTIO PLACENTAE

In abruptio placentae, the placenta separates prematurely from the uterine wall before delivery. Bleeding may be concealed or external. Illustrated here is total abruptio placentae with concealed hemorrhage.

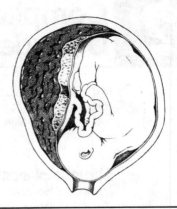

(See also "Disseminated intravascular coagulation" in this section.)

Below is a list of nursing diagnoses and interventions frequently associated with abruptio placentae.

Nursing diagnosis

Altered Peripheral Tissue Perfusion related to hypovolemic shock
Desired outcome: Patient will maintain adequate tissue perfusion.

Nursing interventions and rationales

1. Monitor the patient frequently for signs of shock, checking blood pressure, pulse rate, color, and skin temperature.
Rationale: Hypotension, tachycardia, pallor, and cool, moist skin are indications of hypovolemic shock.
2. Assess and report vaginal bleeding and any increase in fundal height.
Rationale: Increased external or concealed bleeding may be an indication for intervention.
3. Monitor I.V. fluids to help restore circulating fluid volume. Note that an 18G needle should be used.
Rationale: I.V. fluids help maintain circulatory volume and provide a route for rapid administration of blood and fluids, if necessary.
4. Administer oxygen, as ordered (10 to 12 liters/minute by face mask).
Rationale: Oxygen administration increases available oxygen to maternal tissues and organs.
5. Administer blood or blood products as ordered, and observe for reactions.
Rationale: Blood transfusion may be necessary to restore blood volume and maintain tissue perfusion.
6. Monitor the patient's intake and output.
Rationale: Urine production of less than 30 ml/hour may indicate decreased renal perfusion.

Nursing diagnosis

Altered Placental Tissue Perfusion related to inadequate oxygenation

Desired outcome: Adequate placental perfusion and fetal oxygenation will be maintained.

Nursing interventions and rationales

1. Assess the fetal heart rate and fetal monitor pattern.
Rationale: Alterations in placental perfusion decrease fetal oxygenation, resulting in abnormal fetal heart rate response.
2. Encourage the patient to maintain the lateral position.
Rationale: The lateral position provides optimum circulation to the uterus and placenta.
3. Administer oxygen to the patient (10 to 12 liters/minute by face mask), as ordered.
Rationale: Maternal oxygen administration increases available oxygen to the fetus.

Nursing diagnosis

Altered Cardiopulmonary Tissue Perfusion related to hemorrhage secondary to development of DIC

Desired outcome: Patient will maintain normal hemostasis.

Nursing interventions and rationales

1. Observe for abnormal bleeding from needle puncture sites, incisions, and the vagina.
Rationale: Consumption of coagulation factors results in subsequent failure of normal blood-clotting response.
2. Monitor the patient's blood work for signs of impending DIC (low fibrinogen and platelet levels and increased prothrombin time, partial thromboplastin time, blood-clotting time, and fibrin degradation products).
Rationale: Early diagnosis allows for prompt treatment with appropriate blood components.
3. Administer blood and blood components as ordered, and observe for reactions.
Rationale: Transfusions of clotting factors will replace those consumed by the abnormal clotting process in DIC.

Medical diagnosis

Medical diagnosis for abruptio placentae is based on:
• noting clinical objective and subjective data
• using ultrasound to rule out placenta previa (retroplacental clot may be visible in abruptio placentae)
• observing for decreased hemoglobin and hematocrit levels
• noting high baseline uterine tonus with placement of an internal pressure catheter in the uterus.

Medical treatment
Treatment of the patient with abruptio placentae may include:
• hospitalization
• monitoring fetal status and resting uterine tone
• performing early amniotomy (which allows for internal monitoring and may help prevent Couvelaire uterus and DIC by altering intrauterine pressures)
• monitoring clotting factors and hematocrit level
• typing and crossmatching blood
• replacing blood loss to maintain a hematocrit level of 30
• replacing clotting factors as indicated
• using an indwelling (Foley) catheter with hourly output
• inserting a central line for hemodynamic monitoring in critical cases (central venous pressure line or Swan-Ganz pulmonary artery catheter)
• delivering the fetus as quickly as possible (Vaginal delivery is preferable if the fetus is healthy and the patient stable, or if the fetus is dead. Cesarean section is indicated if the fetus is alive but shows signs of distress.)
• performing the Kleihauer-Betke test after delivery for Rh-negative patients because excessive fetal maternal hemorrhage is common with abruptio placentae.

☐ Acquired immunodeficiency syndrome (AIDS)
The human immunodeficiency virus (HIV) is the causative factor in the development of AIDS. The virus attacks lymphocytes and produces immune deficiency by destroying helper T cells, thereby interfering with cell-mediated immunity. The immunocompromised AIDS host is thus susceptible to opportunistic infections and unusual cancers.

The AIDS virus is transmitted by sexual contact with an infected partner, direct inoculation of infected blood products, shared needles during drug use, and perinatal transmission from an infected mother to the fetus or newborn (transplacental transmission, contamination with maternal blood during birth, or through breast milk). Transmission of the virus through artificial insemination with infected semen has also been reported.

Because normal pregnancy involves some suppression of the maternal immune system, it may be during pregnancy that women infected with HIV first demonstrate symptoms of AIDS or possibly develop life-threatening infections. Infants have an immature immune system early in life, and those who become infected with HIV at birth may develop overt disease rapidly.

Predisposing factors include the following:
• history of I.V. drug use

• history of sexual contact with:
  — an I.V. drug user
  — a person with HIV, AIDS, AIDS-related complex, or hemophilia
  — bisexual men
• history of blood transfusion in the United States between 1979 and June 1985 or in an endemic foreign country since 1979
• history of artificial insemination from an infected donor since 1979
• recent immigrants from Haiti or Central Africa or their sexual partners
• multiple sexual partners.
  Frequently encountered data for AIDS include the following:

Subjective data
• gastrointestinal discomfort
• dyspnea or shortness of breath
• arthralgia
• headache, memory loss, or confusion
• fatigue, decreased libido, or depression

Objective data
• enlarged lymph nodes
• recurrent fever or night sweats
• weight loss
• diarrhea
• oral thrush
• cough
• opportunistic infections (*Pneumocystic carinii* pneumonia, toxoplasmosis)
• Kaposi's sarcoma
• enlarged spleen.
  Below is a list of nursing diagnoses and interventions frequently associated with AIDS.

Nursing diagnosis
High Risk for Infection related to suppressed immune response
Desired outcome: Patient will be protected against exposure to infection.

Nursing interventions and rationales
1. Place the patient in protective isolation.
Rationale: This prevents the introduction of infection to the patient.
2. Observe for signs of infection (increased temperature, pulse rate, and white blood cell count).
Rationale: Early diagnosis and prompt treatment will minimize complications.

Nursing diagnosis
High Risk for Injury related to transmission of disease
Desired outcome: Patient will not infect other individuals.

Nursing interventions and rationales
1. Isolate all body fluids.
Rationale: Isolation will remove a potential source of infection to others.
2. Take needle precautions, including wearing gloves and not re-capping needles.
Rationale: Needle sticks represent one of the greatest hazards to medical personnel.
3. Promptly remove the newborn from contact with the mother's blood.
Rationale: Removal eliminates a potential source of infection for the newborn.
4. Restrict breast-feeding.
Rationale: HIV transmission through breast milk has been documented.
5. Educate the patient regarding HIV transmission.
Rationale: HIV-positive patients, especially those who are asymptomatic, have the potential to infect many other people.

Nursing diagnosis
Knowledge Deficit related to AIDS infection and transmission
Desired outcome: Patient will understand modes of transmission and alter her lifestyle to protect others.

Nursing interventions and rationales
1. Stress the necessity of regular medical evaluation and follow-up.
Rationale: Regular medical surveillance and prompt treatment of opportunistic infections may prevent further complications.
2. Urge the patient to refrain from donating blood, plasma, or body organs.
Rationale: All of these are sources of infection for other individuals.
3. Advise the patient to avoid sharing toothbrushes, razors, or other implements potentially contaminated with blood.
Rationale: All of these are sources of infection.
4. Advise the patient to avoid becoming pregnant again.
Rationale: Pregnancy often causes a deterioration in the patient's condition.
5. Instruct the patient to inform doctors, dentists, and all other medical personnel of the diagnosis so that appropriate precautions can be taken.
Rationale: The patient should assume the responsibility of informing others about the infection to avoid transmission.
6. Advise the patient to inform her sexual partners of the diagnosis.

Rationale: All contacts should be tested for HIV.
7. Persuade the patient not to engage in sexual activity that involves the exchange of body fluids.
Rationale: All body fluids are potential sources of infection.

Nursing diagnosis
Anticipatory Grieving related to poor prognosis
Desired outcome: Patient deals with the stages of grief and functions at an adequate level.
Nursing interventions and rationales
1. Provide opportunities for the patient to discuss her feelings and concerns realistically.
Rationale: Verbalization of feelings can be therapeutic and provides insight into the patient's perceptions of her disease.
2. Identify the stages of grieving.
Rationale: Awareness allows for appropriate interventions.
3. Assess the need for referral to other resources, such as counseling, clergy, or support groups.
Rationale: The patient may need additional help to deal with diagnosis and prognosis.

Other nursing diagnoses
This list of additional diagnoses may apply to the AIDS patient:
• Fear related to the nature of the condition and its implications for the patient's lifestyle
• Hopelessness related to the incurable nature of the disease
• Social Isolation related to fear of disease transmission

Medical diagnosis
Medical diagnosis for AIDS patients is based on:
• screening for patients in high-risk groups (see the predisposing factors mentioned above).
• ELISA screening test for the AIDS antibody (Positive tests indicate the need for further testing using the Western blot. These tests are antibody-specific. The patient may be infected with the virus [antigen] but not yet have produced antibodies, thereby testing negative but being capable of infecting others. Repeated testing during the third trimester and 6 months after the initial test is necessary to ensure a negative status—provided the patient has not become infected during that time. Patients infected with the virus may take 2 to 3 months or longer to produce antibodies.)
• Infants born to HIV-positive patients will test positive because the mother's positive antibody may persist for as long as 18 months after birth. (About 30% to 50% of infants born to HIV-positive women will acquire the infection.)

Medical treatment

Treatment for AIDS may include zidovudine (Retrovir) to prevent HIV replication, not a cure for the disease (associated with producing many side effects, the drug is expensive and must be taken every 4 hours around the clock); supportive care; prompt treatment of opportunistic infections.

As a preventive measure, procedures that increase the risk of perinatal transmission, such as chorionic villi sampling, amniocentesis, fetal scalp sampling, should be avoided.

☐ Anemia

Defined as a hemoglobin level below 10 g/dl or a hematocrit level below 30%, anemia is the most common medical disorder of pregnancy, predisposing the patient to postpartum infection and hemorrhage. More than 90% of pregnant patients with anemia develop the disorder as a result of iron deficiency. Hemoglobin and hematocrit values normally drop during pregnancy because of the increased plasma volume, but not to this level.

Predisposing factors include the following:
• multiple gestation
• infection
• pica
• short interpregnancy interval
• poor nutritional status
• failure to take prescribed supplements during pregnancy.

Frequently encountered data for anemia include the following:

Subjective data
• fatigue
• headache

Objective data
• pallor
• systolic heart murmur
• tachycardia
• hemoglobin below 10 g/dl and hematocrit below 30%.

Below is a list of the nursing diagnoses and interventions frequently associated with anemia.

Nursing diagnosis

Impaired Gas Exchange related to altered oxygen-carrying capacity of the blood
Desired outcome: Hemoglobin and hematocrit levels return to acceptable levels to prevent complications during pregnancy.

Nursing interventions and rationales

1. Monitor hemoglobin and hematocrit values every 2 weeks.
Rationale: Patients on iron replacement therapy should begin to show a response after 2 weeks.

2. Instruct the patient to consume foods high in iron and folic acid.
Rationale: Dietary improvement helps restore iron stores.
3. Evaluate the patient's diet for adequate protein intake.
Rationale: Adequate protein in the diet is an important source of iron.
4. Administer iron supplements, as ordered. Instruct the patient to take them with a source of vitamin C and to avoid taking them with tea.
Rationale: Vitamin C aids in the absorption of iron. Tannic acid in tea impedes iron absorption.
5. Educate the client regarding the importance of correcting the anemia to prevent complications.
Rationale: The patient may be unaware of the importance of adequate iron intake.

Nursing diagnosis
Fluid Volume Deficit related to postpartum hemorrhage
Desired outcome: Patient has no significant blood loss at delivery.

Nursing interventions and rationales
1. Instruct the patient in ways to prevent or correct anemia (diet, proper medication). Stress the importance of correcting anemia before the time of labor.
Rationale: Prevention or correction of anemia may help to prevent significant bleeding.
2. Check the patient's hemoglobin and hematocrit levels during labor, when ordered. Note that values may be falsely elevated because of decreased fluid intake.
Rationale: Anticipation of possible bleeding allows for interventions to prevent abnormal blood loss.
3. Monitor the patient closely for abnormal bleeding after delivery.
Rationale: Prompt intervention prevents significant complications.

Nursing diagnosis
High Risk for Infection related to anemia
Desired outcome: Puerperal infection does not occur.

Nursing interventions and rationales
1. Monitor the anemic postpartum patient closely for signs and symptoms of infection.
Rationale: Prompt treatment can prevent further complications.
2. Minimize the patient's risk of developing an infection by observing hospital procedures, such as wearing scrub clothes and washing hands.
Rationale: Many infections are hospital-acquired.

Medical diagnosis

The medical diagnosis for anemia is based on:
• complete blood cell count with erythrocyte indices (hemoglobin and hematocrit levels below 10g/dl and 30%, respectively, with microcytic, hypochromic cells)
• serum iron levels, total iron-binding capacity, and serum ferritin levels. (Patients taking iron supplements may not demonstrate accurate results.)

Medical treatment

Treatment for anemia may include:
• iron and folic acid supplements
• a diet high in iron, protein, and vitamin C
• injectible iron, to be used only in severe cases because the potential side effects are significant (It does not speed the response to therapy.)
• transfusion (rarely necessary)
• administration of oxytocic drugs postpartum to prevent hemorrhage.

☐ Birth trauma

Infant birth trauma can result from the forces of labor; abnormal fetal presentations, positions, or size; resistance of soft tissue or the bony pelvis; or the actual birth. Many injuries are minor and resolve without treatment; some are serious enough to cause permanent damage or death.

Predisposing factors include the following:
• forceps deliveries
• shoulder dystocia
• malpresentations
• use of a vacuum extractor
• macrosomia
• precipitate birth.

Frequently encountered data for birth trauma include the following:

Subjective data
Not applicable

Objective data
• caput succedaneum (localized edema of the scalp)
• cephalohematoma (collection of blood between the periosteum and the bones of the skull; seen more commonly with vacuum extraction)
• scleral and retinal hemorrhages (ruptured capillaries within the eye)
• subcutaneous fat necrosis (firm mass fixed to the overlying skin from pressure against the pelvis or from forceps)

• ecchymoses (bruising anywhere on the body, usually from forceps)
• skull fracture (asymptomatic or with symptoms from increased intracranial pressure; usually a result of difficult delivery or forceps)
• fractured clavicle (limitation of the motion of the arm, crepitus of the bone, and lack of a Moro reflex on the affected side; usually from shoulder dystocia)
• fractures of humerus or femur (lack of movement, abnormal positioning; usually the result of a difficult delivery)
• brachial paralysis, upper arm (Erb-Duchenne paralysis: flaccid arm with the elbow extended and the hand rotated inward; negative Moro reflex on the affected side; usually the result of a difficult delivery)
• brachial paralysis, lower arm (Klumpke's paralysis: flaccid wrist and hand, absent grasp reflex, dependent edema, cyanosis; the consequence of a difficult delivery)
• facial paralysis (face unresponsive to stimulation or to the grimace of crying, with the eye unable to close; usually caused by misapplied forceps)
• intraventricular hemorrhage (caused by trauma, asphyxia, or prematurity).

   Below is a list of nursing diagnoses and interventions frequently associated with birth trauma.

Nursing diagnosis
High Risk for Injury related to tissue damage at birth
Desired outcome: Damage is minimized or does not occur.

Nursing interventions and rationales
1. Perform a complete physical assessment when the newborn is admitted to the nursery.
Rationale: Early diagnosis and intervention can prevent further complications.
2. Implement corrective action as soon as possible after the diagnosis is made.
Rationale: Corrective action prevents more extensive damage.
3. Maintain an observation for the development of symptoms of birth trauma in predisposed infants.
Rationale: Some injuries, such as intraventricular hemorrhage, do not manifest symptoms immediately.

Nursing diagnosis
Altered Parenting related to abnormality in the newborn
Desired outcome: Effective maternal-infant bonding occurs.

Nursing interventions and rationales

1. Explain the injury to the family and provide factual information regarding the prognosis.
Rationale: Keeping the family informed prevents unrealistic fears from developing and helps to allay their anxieties.
2. Allow the parents to interact with the infant to the fullest extent possible depending on the injury.
Rationale: Interaction facilitates maternal-infant attachment.

Medical diagnoses

Medical diagnosis for birth trauma is based on clinical presentation, X-ray to diagnose fractures, and computed tomography scan to diagnose intraventricular hemorrhage.

Medical treatment

Prevention is the key. The following treatments pertain only to those conditions that require medical intervention:
• for fractured humerus or femur: slings, splints to immobilize the extremity while it is healing
• for brachial paralysis: intermittent immobilization, proper positioning, and exercise to maintain range of motion
• for facial paralysis: careful feeding and preventing damage to the cornea
• for intraventricular hemorrhage: serial lumbar punctures, diuretics, osmotic agents; shunt placement for unresponsive cases.

☐ Breech presentation

Breech presentations carry a higher rate of neonatal morbidity than cephalic presentations (see *Examples of breech presentation*). Prolapse of the cord, entrapment of the after-coming head by the cervix, cephalopelvic disproportion, and birth trauma are all potential complications of breech presentations. A steady trend toward delivery by cesarean section for all breech presentations has been developing. Recently, the technique of external version has been reintroduced to decrease the incidence of breech presentations at term (see "External version" in Section 3).
 Predisposing factors include the following:
• previous breech presentations
• uterine anomalies
• placenta previa
• hydrocephalus
• multiple gestation
• prematurity
• high parity
• anencephalus
• tumors of the uterus
• polyhydramnios or oligohydramnios.

EXAMPLES OF BREECH PRESENTATION

In a breech presentation, the buttocks face downward in the birth canal, as illustrated here.

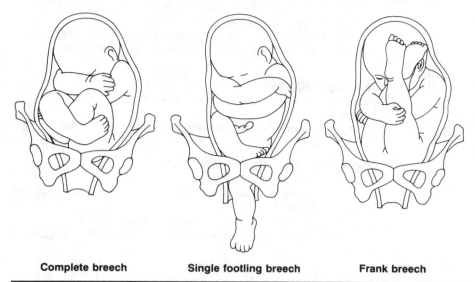

| Complete breech | Single footling breech | Frank breech |

Frequently encountered data for breech presentation include the following:

Subjective data
• fetal activity concentrated below the umbilicus

Objective data
• fetal head palpated in the fundus
• fetal heart tones above the umbilicus
• passage of thick meconium in labor (not related to fetal distress)
• breech palpated by vaginal examination.

Below is a list of nursing diagnoses and interventions frequently associated with breech presentations.

Nursing diagnosis

High Risk for Injury related to decreased oxygenation secondary to prolapsed cord, cord compression, or entrapment of the head
Desired outcome: Fetus maintains adequate oxygenation during labor and delivery.

Nursing interventions and rationales

1. Maintain fetal monitoring throughout labor.
Rationale: This enables early detection of abnormal fetal heart rates.
2. Avoid early rupture of the membranes, if possible.

Rationale: Amniotic fluid acts as a cushion for the cord; the cord cannot prolapse while the membranes are intact.

3. Check fetal heart tones immediately after rupture of the membranes, and perform a vaginal examination.

Rationale: Early diagnosis of prolapsed cord allows for prompt intervention, which minimizes the incidence of permanent injury.

Nursing diagnosis

High Risk for Injury related to exhaustion secondary to prolonged labor

Desired outcome: The nurse recognizes and reports signs of dysfunctional labor.

Nursing interventions and rationales

1. Monitor uterine activity.

Rationale: Monitoring uterine activity is important for evaluating the progression of labor.

2. Monitor cervical changes and station of the breech.

Rationale: Monitoring is important for evaluating the progression of labor.

Nursing diagnosis

Fear related to possible fetal injury from breech presentation

Desired outcome: Client verbalizes feelings and the reason for the plan of care.

Nursing interventions and rationales

1. Keep the patient and her family informed of the labor's progress and plan of care.

Rationale: Knowledge of the labor's progress and of the plan of care will lessen anxiety.

2. Reassure the patient as needed (show her the fetal monitor strip if it is normal).

Rationale: Such reassurance lessens fear.

Medical diagnosis

Medical diagnosis for breech presentation is based on:
• vaginal examination
• ultrasound examination
• abdominal X-ray.

Medical treatment

Treatment may include:
• external version, which can be attempted if the patient is not in labor and if the breech is not engaged
• delivery by cesarean section (indicated for a primigravida with a breech presentation or for patients with footling or complete breech presentations)

• vaginal delivery (usually reserved for patients with frank breech presentation). The following measures should be taken:
  — assessing for fetal weight and pelvic size
  — X-ray pelvimetry to determine attitude of fetal head (must be flexed on the chest)
  — fetal monitoring throughout labor
  — fetal scalp blood sampling to assess for fetal distress in the presence of abnormal fetal heart rate patterns
  — delaying the rupture of membranes, if possible
  — liberal use of cesarean section for dysfunctional labor.

(*Note:* Oxytocin use is controversial with breech presentations.)

☐ Cesarean section

The removal of the fetus from the uterus through an incision made into the abdominal wall and uterus, cesarean section can be categorized as primary, repeat, or elective. Primary cesarean section refers to the patient's initial experience with this type of delivery. Repeat cesarean section refers to any subsequent abdominal deliveries. Elective cesarean section is one that is planned and performed before the onset of labor.

Several incision sites are available; the two most common are the classical (vertical) and the low-segment (bikini) incision. However, the low-segment type is preferred because it involves less blood loss and because the incision on the uterus is less likely to rupture during subsequent pregnancies; the lower segment contains fewer contractile fibers than the fundus.

The possibility of vaginal birth after cesarean section (VBAC) has gained popularity among health care providers and mothers; low-segment incision is usually required for this procedure (see "Vaginal birth after cesarean section" in Section 3).

Maternal mortality is four times higher with cesarean section than with vaginal delivery. Maternal morbidity is also increased because of infections of the uterus, urinary tract, or lungs and because of hemorrhage. Prematurity is the most common complication for the newborn, as a result of misjudgment of the duration of gestation. Transient tachypnea of the newborn is usually a result of retained secretions in the respiratory tract. (See "Preterm birth" and "Transient tachypnea of the newborn" in this section.)

Predisposing factors include the following:
• previous cesarean section
• breech presentation
• transverse lie
• placenta previa
• fetal distress
• dysfunctional labor
• cephalopelvic disproportion
• severe pregnancy-induced hypertension (PIH)

- abruptio placentae
- prolapsed cord
- active maternal herpes
- invasive cancer of the cervix
- hydrocephaly
- multiple gestation.

For frequently encountered data for cesarean section, refer to the predisposing factors listed above. Below is a list of nursing diagnoses and interventions frequently associated with cesarean section. (See the predisposing factors listed above as well as those for "Preterm labor" and "Transient tachypnea of the newborn" in this section.)

Nursing diagnosis

Fear related to the indications for cesarean section and possible complications for mother or infant
Desired outcome: Patient verbalizes her fears and accepts the reason for operative intervention.

Nursing interventions and rationales

1. Explain the indication for the patient's cesarean section and provide appropriate reassurance regarding its outcome.
Rationale: The patient may have unrealistic fears about the procedure and outcome.
2. Provide preoperative teaching.
Rationale: Preoperative teaching helps to prepare the patient for what to expect postoperatively.

Nursing diagnosis

Pain related to surgical incision
Desired outcome: Patient verbalizes relief from pain within an acceptable period of time after experiencing the pain.

Nursing interventions and rationales

1. Monitor the patient's level of comfort frequently.
Rationale: Providing pain relief before the pain becomes severe may provide more effective analgesia.
2. Evaluate the patient's response to analgesic drugs.
Rationale: Some patients require different dosages or changing to a different medication.
3. Provide other comfort measures as appropriate (back rub, position change).
Rationale: Use of other stimuli can decrease the level of pain.

Nursing diagnosis

High Risk for Injury related to complications from surgery (infection, hemorrhage, thromboembolism)
Desired outcome: Patient has no postoperative complications.

Nursing interventions and rationales
1. Monitor the patient's vital signs closely.
Rationale: Decreased blood pressure, increased pulse rate, and increased temperature are signs of infection or blood loss. (See also "Postpartum hemorrhage" in this section.)
2. Observe for signs and symptoms of complications.
Rationale: Burning and pain on urination may indicate bladder infection. Tender uterus and foul-smelling lochia are signs of endometritis. Productive cough or chills may indicate pneumonia. Positive Homans' sign, pain, or edema of an extremity may indicate thrombophlebitis.
3. Use sterile technique (for dressing changes); encourage the patient to turn, cough, and deep breathe, and to ambulate early.
Rationale: These interventions prevent infection, pneumonia, and thromboembolism.

Nursing diagnosis
High Risk for Altered Parenting related to operative delivery
Desired outcome: Effective maternal-infant bonding occurs.

Nursing interventions and rationales
1. Recommend that a regional anesthetic be used, if possible.
Rationale: Regional anesthetics allow the patient to remain awake so she can interact with her newborn immediately.
2. Provide the earliest possible opportunity for parents to see, hold, and touch the newborn.
Rationale: Early interaction facilitates attachment.
3. Provide the parents with an opportunity to explore their feelings regarding cesarean section delivery.
Rationale: Feelings of guilt, regret, loss, and failure can interfere with the normal postpartum course.

Medical diagnosis
Medical diagnosis for cesarean section is based on:
• confirmed diagnosis of any of the predisposing factors listed above
• determination of fetal maturity, using ultrasound or amniocentesis for the lecithin-sphingomyelin ratio (should be done before cesarean section unless an emergency precludes such testing).

Medical treatment
Treatment for cesarean section may include:
• treatment related to any of the predisposing factors listed above
• at least 2 units of whole blood (typed and crossmatched)
• insertion of an indwelling (Foley) catheter
• administration of an antacid, such as sodium citrate, before surgery; this may help to minimize the risk of lung destruction from gastric hydrochloric acid if aspiration occurs

• administration of I.V. fluids; oxytocin is added after the infant is delivered
• administration of analgesics for postoperative pain
• progressive postoperative care similar to that for other abdominal surgeries.

☐ Chorioamnionitis

A bacterial infection of the amniotic cavity, chorioamnionitis is a significant cause of perinatal mortality and maternal morbidity. It occurs most commonly after rupture of the membranes; however, it can also occur with intact membranes. It has been well correlated with the subsequent development of premature labor.

Chorioamnionitis may lead to the development of postpartum endometritis, which is most common in patients who deliver by cesarean section. Perinatal mortality is especially increased among premature infants. Neonatal morbidity from sepsis and its complications is also significant.

Predisposing factors include the following:
• premature rupture of the membranes (PROM)
• vaginitis
• amniocentesis
• intrauterine procedures.

Frequently encountered data for chorioamnionitis include the following:

Subjective data
• uterine tenderness
• uterine contractions

Objective data
• elevated temperature
• maternal and/or fetal tachycardia
• foul odor to the amniotic fluid
• leukocytosis
• uterine activity.

Below is a list of nursing diagnoses and interventions frequently associated with chorioamnionitis. (See also "Dystocia," "Endometritis," "Postpartum hemorrhage," and "Sepsis" in this section.)

Nursing diagnosis

High Risk for Injury to Mother, Fetus, or Newborn related to chorioamnionitis
Desired outcome: No complications occur in the mother, fetus, or newborn.

Nursing interventions and rationales

1. Monitor vital signs frequently.

Rationale: Alterations in vital signs may be one of earliest signs of impending complications.

2. Observe the fetal monitoring strip for a change in the fetal heart pattern.

Rationale: Fetal distress is a common result of the infectious process and of umbilical cord compression (which is brought about by ruptured membranes).

3. Monitor uterine activity for dysfunctional labor pattern.

Rationale: Dysfunctional labor is common and can be treated with a trial of oxytocin augmentation. Labor should not be prolonged because of increased maternal and neonatal morbidity.

Nursing diagnosis
Fear related to diagnosis and the possibility of complications in the mother or newborn

Desired outcome: Patient verbalizes her fears and an understanding of the plan of care.

Nursing interventions and rationales
1. Assess the patient's understanding of the diagnosis and plan of care.

Rationale: The nurse can identify individual needs of the patient.

2. Discuss with the patient the plan of care, explaining its rationale and allowing her to ask questions.

Rationale: Understanding the situation and the reason for intervention alleviates fear of the unknown.

3. Allow the support person to remain with the patient as much as possible.

Rationale: The presence of a person the patient knows well and trusts is reassuring.

Medical diagnosis
Medical diagnosis for chorioamnionitis is based on:
• documentation of clinical signs and symptoms
• blood culture
• amniotic fluid analysis (by amniocentesis) for Gram stain and leukocyte count.

Medical treatment
Treatment for chorioamnionitis includes:
• delivery of the fetus as soon as possible after the diagnosis is made (If a long labor is anticipated, cesarean section may be preferred. Labor often becomes dysfunctional as a result of the infectious process. Patients presenting in preterm labor with intact membranes may have chorioamnionitis. These patients tend to be very resistant to tocolytic therapy; tocolytic drugs should be used with caution.)

• delaying antibiotic treatment until after delivery to improve the accuracy of neonatal cultures (Some health care providers recommend immediate use of antibiotics to limit maternal sepsis and to initiate therapy for the fetus.)
• increasing postpartum uterine tone with oxytocic agents (after delivery to prevent significant blood loss).

☐ Congenital anomalies

Structural defects present at birth, congenital anomalies result from abnormal tissue differentiation or abnormal tissue organ interaction during fetal development. Approximately 10% of congenital anomalies are environmentally caused by exposure to teratogenic agents.

Predisposing factors include the following:
• chromosomal or genetic abnormalities
• exposure to teratogenic agents, such as radiation, drugs, and alcohol, during pregnancy (see *Teratogens and their effects on the fetus,* pages 77 to 79)
• maternal disease (diabetes, epilepsy, infections).

Frequently encountered data for congenital anomalies include the following:

Subjective data
Usually none

Objective data
• abnormal fetal position (breech)
• abnormal growth in fundal height (Growth retardation, oligohydramnios, and polyhydramnios commonly are associated with congenital anomalies.)
• abnormal fetal heart rate or rhythm (congenital heart defects)
• abnormality seen on ultrasound
• abnormal karyotype obtained from cells from amniocentesis or chorionic villi sampling
• abnormality noted at birth during the physical assessment or from signs and symptoms that develop after delivery.

Below is a list of nursing diagnoses and interventions frequently associated with congenital anomalies. (Nursing diagnoses associated with specific anomalies will not be included.)

Nursing diagnosis

High Risk for Altered Parenting related to the birth of an infant with a congenital anomaly
Desired outcome: Parents are able to bond effectively with their infant.

Nursing interventions and rationales

1. Allow the parents to see their baby as soon as possible.

TERATOGENS AND THEIR EFFECTS ON THE FETUS

Agent	Effect	Comments
CHEMICALS AND DRUGS		
Alcohol	Intrauterine growth retardation, mental retardation, fetal alcohol syndrome (including maxillary hypoplasia, prominence of the mandible and forehead, short palpebral fissures, microphthalmos, epicanthal folds, and microcephaly)	• Ingestion of one or two drinks per day (1 to 2 oz) may cause small reductions in the average birth weight. • Ingestion of six drinks per day (6 oz) places the fetus at a 40% risk of developing some of the characteristic features of fetal alcohol syndrome.
Androgens	Pseudohermaphroditism in females, advanced genital development in males	• Effects depend on the drug dosage and stage of embryonic development. • Depending on the length of the fetus' exposure to the drug, clitoral enlargement or labioscrotal fusion may occur. • Brief exposure to the drug produces minimal risks to the fetus.
Anticoagulants (dicumarol, warfarin)	Intrauterine growth retardation; hypoplastic nose; ophthalmologic abnormalities; neck anomalies; defects of the central nervous system (CNS); stippling of the secondary epiphyses; broad, short hands with shortened fingers	• Use of vitamin K-inhibiting anticoagulants during the first trimester places the fetus at a 25% risk of developing serious defects. • Exposure to the drug during the second or third trimester may cause spontaneous abortion, stillbirth, CNS abnormalities, abruptio placentae, or fetal or newborn hemorrhaging.
Antineoplastics (methotrexate)	Increased risk for spontaneous abortion, other fetal anomalies	• These drugs are usually contraindicated for treating psoriasis during pregnancy; they should be used with extreme caution when used to treat cancer. • Use of aminopterin or methotrexate during the first trimester places the fetus at a 30% risk of developing anomalies should he survive.
Diethylstilbestrol (DES)	Cervical and uterine abnormalities, vaginal adenosis, possible infertility (for males and females)	• Use of this drug before the 9th week of pregnancy places the female fetus at a 50% risk of developing vaginal adenosis. • Fetal exposure places males at a 25% risk of developing epididymal cysts, hypotrophic testes, abnormal spermatozoa, or induration of the testes.
Isotretinoin	Increased abortion rate, microtia, CNS defects, cardiovascular system defects, craniofacial defects, microphthalmos, cleft palate	• Because this drug is considered one of the most potent teratogens, its use during pregnancy is contraindicated. If conception should occur during therapy, strong consideration should be given to terminating the pregnancy.

(continued)

TERATOGENS AND THEIR EFFECTS ON THE FETUS *(continued)*

Agent	Effect	Comments
CHEMICALS AND DRUGS (continued)		
Lead	Increased abortion rate, stillbirth	• Lead exposure during pregnancy may cause adverse CNS effects.
Lithium	Congenital heart disease (particularly Ebstein's anomaly)	• Use of this drug during the first trimester places the fetus at a 2% risk of developing heart defects. • Fetal exposure during the last month of pregnancy may have toxic effects on the kidneys, thyroid, and neuromuscular system.
Organic mercury	Mental retardation, cerebral atrophy, blindness, seizures, spasticity	• Fetal exposure, even as late as the third trimester, may cause cerebral palsy. • Exposure usually results from ingestion of grain or fish contaminated with methyl mercury.
Phenytoin	Fetal hydantoin syndrome (including facial abnormalities and anomalies of the fingers and toes), growth deficiency, mental retardation, microcephaly	• Less than 10% of fetuses exposed in utero develop full fetal hydantoin syndrome; however, up to 30% have some manifestations. • About two thirds of those with severe physical defects also have mild to moderate mental retardation.
Streptomycin	Hearing loss, damage to cranial nerve VIII	• Studies with animals have indicated exposure to this drug causes histologic changes to the inner ear.
Tetracycline	Hypoplasia of tooth enamel, incorporation of tetracycline into the bone	• Effects result from fetal exposure during the second or third trimester.
Thalidomide	Bilateral limb deficiencies, anotia, and microtia	• The incidence of adverse effects from fetal exposure to this drug is 20%.
Thyroid hormone antagonists (iodide, methimazole, propylthiouracil)	Hypothyroidism, fetal goiter	• Effects usually depend on the dosage and length of exposure to the drug. • Fetal goiter may lead to malpresentation with hyperextension of the head.
Trimethadione, paramethadione	Cleft lip or palate, cardiac defects, intrauterine growth retardation, microcephaly, mental retardation, ophthalmologic anomalies, fetal trimethadione syndrome (including V-shaped eyebrows, low-set ears, high arched palate, and irregular teeth)	• Exposure to the drug during the first trimester places the fetus at a 60% to 80% risk of spontaneous abortion.

TERATOGENS AND THEIR EFFECTS ON THE FETUS *(continued)*

Agent	Effect	Comments
CHEMICALS AND DRUGS (continued)		
Valproic acid	Neural tube defects	• The incidence of neural tube defects in exposed fetuses is 1% to 2%. • Open-tube defects are caused by fetal exposure to the drug during the first trimester before normal closure of the neural tube occurs.
INFECTIONS		
Cytomegalovirus (CMV)	Microcephaly, somatic growth retardation, brain damage, hearing loss	• Although 0.5% to 1.5% of newborns exposed to the virus have CMV colonization, only 0.1% have severe defects.
Rubella	Heart lesions, cataracts, deafness, other anomalies associated with congenital rubella syndrome	• With maternal infection during the first trimester, the fetal malformation rate is 50%; this rate decreases to 6% by midterm. • Immunization, necessary for prevention of the virus, is contraindicated during pregnancy, although the vaccine virus has not been reported to cause the malformations associated with congenital rubella syndrome.
Syphilis	With severe infection, fetal death caused by edema; with mild infection, abnormalities of the skin, teeth, and bones	• Penicillin therapy effectively destroys the infecting organism (*Treponema pallidum*), thus halting the progression of fetal damage, the severity of which depends on the duration of fetal exposure to the infection.
Toxoplasmosis	Possible effects on all organs	• The severity of effects depend on the duration of the infection, which must be contracted maternally during pregnancy to place the fetus at risk. • The incidence of fetal infection is 15% during the first trimester, increasing to 75% in the third trimester; however, the severity of infection is greater during the first trimester than at the end of pregnancy.
Varicella	Possible effects on all organs, including scarring of the skin and muscle atrophy	• The incidence of congenital varicella is relatively low. • If the newborn was exposed in utero during the last few days of pregnancy, zoster immune globulin may be given.
RADIATION		
X-ray therapy	Mental retardation, microcephaly	• Radiation exposure for medical diagnosis (less than 10 radiation absorbed dose) poses little or no teratogenic risk to the fetus.

Adapted from American College of Obstetricians and Gynecologists. "Teratology," *ACOG Technical Bulletin* 84:1-2, February 1985.

Rationale: Early contact facilitates attachment.

2. Show and explain the defect to the parents, but also focus on the normal aspects of the infant.

Rationale: Presenting the situation realistically, but in perspective, allows the parents to see the anomaly as well as the normal aspects of the infant.

3. Provide factual information regarding the infant's diagnosis and prognosis. (Usually provided by a geneticist or doctor, this information may not be immediately available.)

Rationale: This information may help the parents to realistically face the impact the anomaly will have on them and their child. It may provide a solid basis on which they can dispel any unrealistic hopes and fears.

4. Provide additional support, such as clergy or parent support groups, as needed.

Rationale: Parents frequently need additional support at this time.

5. Accept the parents' reactions and behaviors.

Rationale: The initial reaction may be one of rejection. Give the parents time alone to work through their feelings.

Nursing diagnosis

Self-Esteem Disturbance related to the birth of a child with a congenital anomaly

Desired outcome: Patient and partner express positive feelings about themselves.

Nursing interventions and rationales

1. Encourage the parents to express feelings about producing a child with a congenital anomaly.

Rationale: Verbalization of feelings is therapeutic and provides the nurse with information regarding the family's need for additional support and counseling.

2. Provide information regarding the known etiology of the specific anomaly.

Rationale: Understanding the etiology of the anomaly may help the parents to avoid unfounded anger and self-blame.

3. Refer the parents for professional counseling if you observe strong evidence of guilt or blame.

Rationale: The family may require counseling beyond the scope of what the nurse can provide.

Nursing diagnosis

Fear related to uncertain prognosis and anticipation of physical care for the infant

Desired outcome: Patient verbalizes her feelings and is able to cope with the care the infant requires.

Nursing interventions and rationales

1. Allow the patient time to verbalize her feelings.

Rationale: Verbalization is therapeutic and serves as a source of information for the nurse regarding the patient's need for support, counseling, and teaching.

2. Provide information regarding the infant's prognosis.

Rationale: Information regarding the prognosis may prevent unrealistic ideas about the future and may help the family to begin working through their feelings.

3. Involve support groups as indicated.

Rationale: Contact with other parents who are successfully coping with the same situation can be helpful.

4. Allow the patient adequate time to assume responsibility for caring for her infant.

Rationale: Some anomalies require specialized physical care that can be overwhelming for parents.

Medical diagnosis

Medical diagnosis for congenital anomalies is based on:
• genetic counseling
• chorionic villi sampling (see "Chorionic villi sampling" in Section 3)
• amniocentesis (see "Amniocentesis" in Section 3)
• ultrasound
• maternal serum alpha-fetoprotein (MSAFP plus) studies
• screening of newborns for inborn metabolic errors.

Medical treatment

Treatment of congenital anomalies includes the following (note that specific anomalies will not be included):
• optional termination of pregnancy because of abnormalities indicated by testing
• amniocentesis to determine if the anomaly is compatible with extrauterine life (This procedure should be performed for patients showing fetal abnormalities on ultrasound after abortion is no longer an option. Fetuses with such anomalies frequently develop significant distress during labor, resulting in the need for cesarean section. If the anomalies are known to be incompatible with life, the patient can be spared unnecessary surgery.)
• fetal treatment in utero or fetal surgery (available for some anomalies)
• early delivery and/or delivery by cesarean section (may be indicated for some anomalies, including hydrocephalus, myelomeningocele, and teratomas).

☐ Diabetes mellitus

Pregnancy places special demands on carbohydrate metabolism and causes insulin requirements to increase, even in otherwise healthy patients. It may lead to development of gestational diabetes in previously healthy patients or to complications in previously stable diabetic patients. This discussion will focus on insulin-dependent and gestational diabetes.

Insulin-dependent diabetes

During pregnancy, maternal glucose crosses the placenta; however, insulin does not. The fetus, capable of producing his or her own insulin in response to fluctuating glucose levels, siphons glucose from the mother during the first trimester, causing maternal insulin needs to decrease. This, coupled with the nausea and vomiting of early pregnancy, predisposes the insulin-dependent diabetic to hypoglycemic reactions.

During the second and third trimesters, progressive increases in placental hormones (human placental lactogen, estrogen, progesterone, insulinase, cortisol) cause an insulin-resistant state that necessitates increasing the patient's insulin dosage as the pregnancy progresses. After the placenta is delivered, placental hormone levels drop abruptly and insulin requirements decrease markedly.

Gestational diabetes

Occurring during the second or third trimester, gestational (or chemical) diabetes manifests itself in patients not previously diagnosed as diabetic when the pancreas cannot respond to the demand for more insulin as the pregnancy progresses.

Gestational diabetes frequently can be treated by diet alone. However, insulin therapy is required in about 10% to 15% of patients. Most gestational diabetics revert to normal after delivery but have an increased risk of developing overt diabetes in their lifetime. Oral hypoglycemic agents are never used in pregnancy.

Pregnant diabetics are at increased risk for pregnancy-induced hypertension (PIH), polyhydramnios, fetal death, macrosomia, spontaneous abortion, congenital anomalies, and respiratory distress in the neonate. Maternal mortality in pregnancy is rare unless ketoacidosis develops; then, the rate may be as high as 5% to 15%. Perinatal mortality is four to five times higher than in normal pregnancies.

Predisposing factors to developing diabetes during pregnancy include the following:
• age over 35
• obesity
• multiple gestation
• family history of diabetes.

Frequently encountered data for diabetes mellitus include the following:

Subjective data
• excessive thirst
• hunger

- frequent urination
- blurred vision
- orthostatic dizziness

Objective data
- glycosuria
- ketonuria
- polyhydramnios
- fetus that is large for gestational age
- signs of PIH
- recurrent urinary tract infections
- recurrent vaginal yeast infections
- weight loss.

    Below is a list of nursing diagnoses and interventions frequently associated with diabetes mellitus.

Nursing diagnosis

High Risk for Injury to Mother, Fetus, or Newborn related to poor control of diabetes during pregnancy
Desired outcome: Patient will maintain normal glucose control during pregnancy. Newborn will not incur anomalies or injuries.

Nursing interventions and rationales

1. Provide preconceptual counseling for all diabetic women to establish normal glucose levels before conception.
Rationale: Poor diabetic control in the first trimester is associated with an increase in congenital anomalies.
2. Screen all patients between the 24th and 28th week of pregnancy for the development of gestational diabetes, as ordered.
Rationale: Early recognition of diabetes in pregnancy is essential to preventing complications.
3. Instruct the patient in following the American Diabetes Association diet, or refer her for nutritional counseling.
Rationale: Following a diabetic diet is essential to maintain normal blood glucose levels and allow for adequate fetal growth. This usually includes 2,000 to 2,400 calories/day or 35 calories for every kilogram of ideal body weight.
4. Check fasting plasma glucose (fasting blood sugar) and 2-hour postprandial plasma glucose (2-hour postprandial blood sugar) levels, as ordered, to monitor diabetic control.
Rationale: The fasting blood sugar level should remain less than 100 mg/dl; the 2-hour postprandial blood sugar level, less than 120 mg/dl for optimum outcome (plasma values).
5. Monitor the patient's urine for ketones.
Rationale: Ketonuria is indicative of either insufficient insulin administration or inadequate food intake. Ketones are not tolerated well by the fetus.
6. Administer insulin, as ordered.
Rationale: Insulin is necessary for the use of glucose by cells. If

the patient has not taken insulin before, she should be given human insulin.

7. Observe the patient for signs and symptoms of hypoglycemia or hyperglycemia.
Rationale: Prompt treatment of abnormal glucose levels will minimize complications.

8. Administer skim milk rather than orange juice for hypoglycemic reactions.
Rationale: Milk will elevate blood glucose levels gradually, whereas juices tend to cause wide fluctuations that are undesirable.

9. Monitor fundal height and sonograms for evidence of excessive fetal growth, polyhydramnios, or anomalies.
Rationale: Hyperglycemia can cause excessive fetal growth. Polyhydramnios and congenital anomalies are more likely to develop with diabetic pregnancies than with nondiabetic pregnancies.

10. Monitor closely for signs of dysfunctional labor and cephalopelvic disproportion.
Rationale: Macrosomatic infants are at increased risk for injury if delivered vaginally.

11. Monitor the newborn for hypoglycemia (blood glucose concentration of less than 30 mg/dl in term infants or less than 20 mg/dl for preterm infants).
Rationale: Maternal glucose readily crosses the placenta, whereas insulin does not. The fetus responds by increasing insulin production. After delivery, the infant is no longer exposed to maternal hyperglycemia; however, the pancreas continues to produce increased amounts of insulin for some time, causing hypoglycemia.

Nursing diagnosis
Altered Placental Tissue Perfusion related to inadequate oxygenation
Desired outcome: Patient will deliver a healthy infant.

Nursing interventions and rationales
1. Monitor the fetal heart rate, fetal activity, and results of fetal surveillance tests (nonstress test, contraction stress test, or biophysical profile weekly or twice a week).
Rationale: Alterations in placental perfusion may decrease activity and cause abnormal fetal heart rate response.

2. Observe for declining insulin needs during the third trimester (hypoglycemic reactions, consistent need to decrease insulin dose).
Rationale: Insulin needs should rise as pregnancy progresses because of increased placental production of hormones that cause increasing insulin resistance.

3. Encourage the patient to maintain the lateral position while in bed.

Rationale: The lateral position provides optimum circulation to the uterus and placenta.

Nursing diagnosis

Knowledge Deficit related to diabetic care and the effect of diabetes on pregnancy
Desired outcome: Patient will develop independence in diabetic care and will verbalize an understanding of the reason for medical treatment.

Nursing interventions and rationales

1. Explain to the patient the metabolic changes of pregnancy and their effect on diabetic control.
Rationale: Understanding the effect of pregnancy on diabetes will help the patient to accept frequent changes in insulin requirements.
2. Review with the patient the prescribed diet, or request nutritional consultation.
Rationale: A thorough understanding of the American Diabetic Association diet is essential for good control.
3. Teach or review the technique for insulin administration.
Rationale: Accurate administration of prescribed insulin and proper rotation of sites are necessary to prevent complications.
4. Instruct the patient in blood glucose monitoring and checking urine for ketones.
Rationale: Many patients check their own glucose levels at home and monitor urine for ketones between office visits.
5. Review with the patient the signs and symptoms of diabetic complications.
Rationale: Prompt recognition and treatment of symptoms can prevent complications.

Nursing diagnosis

High Risk for Infection related to diabetic state
Desired outcome: Patient will develop no concurrent infections during pregnancy or the postpartum period.

Nursing interventions and rationales

1. Observe for general signs and symptoms of infection (increased temperature, pulse rate, and white blood cell count).
Rationale: Early recognition of infection allows for prompt treatment and can prevent more serious complications, such as ketoacidosis.
2. Monitor for signs and symptoms of urinary tract infection (UTI), including burning and pain with urination, lower abdominal pain, hematuria, chills, frequent urination, and positive urine culture.
Rationale: Pregnancy predisposes the patient to the development

of UTIs; the high glucose content of the diabetic patient's urine increases the incidence of infection. Untreated infections can lead to pyelonephritis, which can precipitate premature labor.
3. Monitor for signs of candidal vaginitis, including white, curdy discharge and vaginal itching.
Rationale: Candidal vaginitis occurs more commonly in pregnant women and diabetics. Untreated candidiasis (moniliasis) can cause thrush in the neonate.
4. Monitor for signs of postpartum infection; signs may include engorged, painful breasts, uterine tenderness, or foul-smelling lochia.
Rationale: Diabetic women remain at risk for infection in the postpartum period.

Medical diagnosis
Medical diagnosis for gestational diabetes mellitus is based on:
• diabetic screening for all patients between the 24th and 28th week of pregnancy: 50-g glucose load given at random (patient need not be fasting) with 1-hour plasma glucose level greater than 135 mg/dl indicates a need for glucose tolerance test
• glucose tolerance test (3-hour test, using 100 g of glucose): patient should take in at least 100 g of carbohydrate each day for 3 days before the test; a diagnosis of abnormal glucose tolerance in pregnancy is indicated by an elevated fasting level or if two or more of the following values are met or exceeded:

Fasting (plasma)	105 mg/dl
1-hour test	190 mg/dl
2-hour test	165 mg/dl
3-hour test	145 mg/dl

Medical treatment
Treatment for diabetes mellitus includes:
• following the recommended ADA diet (ingesting approximately 2,000 to 2,400 calories/day or 35 calories/kg of ideal body weight/day)
• insulin therapy if the fasting blood sugar levels are greater than 100 mg/dl or the 2-hour postprandial levels are greater than 120 mg/dl; insulin dosage should be adjusted to maintain levels below these values. Human insulin should be administered to gestational diabetics who have never taken insulin before.
• monitoring hemoglobin A_{1c} levels to evaluate blood glucose levels over the previous 4 to 6 weeks
• fetal surveillance testing (nonstress test, contraction stress test, or biophysical profile) weekly or twice a week beginning at the 28th week (Note that gestational diabetics may be allowed to go to term as long as fetal surveillance testing indicates a healthy fetus.)
• serial sonograms for anomalies, fetal growth, and polyhydramnios

• maternal serum alpha-fetoprotein studies (the incidence of neural tube defects is increased in diabetic pregnancies)
• evaluating the effect of diabetes on maternal systems with ECGs, ophthalmologic examinations, and evaluation of renal function (blood urea nitrogen and serum creatinine levels, creatinine clearance)
• obtaining periodic urine cultures for asymptomatic bacteruria
• amniocentesis at the 37th or 38th week for fetal lung maturity to determine optimal time of delivery for insulin-dependent patients (Lecithin-sphingomyelin ratio of 2:1 cannot be used as a measure of fetal lung maturity in insulin-dependent diabetic pregnancies. The presence of phosphatidylglycerol in amniotic fluid is a more reliable predictor of normal neonatal respiratory function.)
• repeated 3-hour glucose tolerance test at 6 weeks postpartum for gestational diabetics to ensure a return to normal glucose tolerance.

☐ Disseminated intravascular coagulation (DIC)

Occurring in 1 out of every 500 deliveries, DIC is a pathologic syndrome in which clotting is overstimulated throughout the circulatory system by an underlying disease process. This disease process acts on the clotting mechanisms to increase the formation of clots in the microcirculation.

The rapid and extensive formation of clots causes platelets and clotting factors to be depleted. Extensive clotting stimulates the fibrinolytic system to dissolve the clots of fibrin, leading to the formation of fibrin degradation products (fibrin split products), which have an anticoagulant effect. The overall result is frank bleeding and potential vascular occlusion of organs resulting from thromboembolus formation.

Predisposing factors include the following:
• abruptio placentae
• pregnancy-induced hypertension
• intrauterine fetal death
• amniotic fluid embolism
• intra-amniotic injection of saline solution
• hemorrhagic shock
• liver disease
• sepsis.

Frequently encountered data for DIC include the following:

Subjective data
Usually none

Objective data
• bleeding from mucous membranes, I.V. sites, injection sites, and surgical incision

• bruising, purpura, petechiae, and ecchymoses
• occult blood in stool
• hematuria, hematemesis, or vaginal bleeding
• abnormal blood-clotting studies
• low hematocrit level
• restlessness or tachycardia.

Below is a list of the nursing diagnoses and interventions frequently associated with DIC.

Nursing diagnosis
Fluid Volume Deficit related to hemorrhage
Desired outcome: Patient will maintain adequate tissue perfusion.

Nursing interventions and rationales
1. Record the patient's vital signs, and assess for signs of shock every 15 minutes.
Rationale: Profuse bleeding from DIC can rapidly lead to shock. Replacing fluids as quickly as they are lost is often difficult; shock develops even with treatment.
2. Administer blood and blood products as ordered, and observe for a reaction.
Rationale: Blood transfusions will help to restore circulating volume; specific blood products will replace necessary clotting factors.
3. Administer oxygen, as ordered (10 to 12 liters/minute by face mask).
Rationale: Oxygen administration increases available oxygen to maternal organs and tissues.

Nursing diagnosis
High Risk for Altered Parenting related to ineffective bonding secondary to disease (DIC)
Desired outcome: Parents will bond effectively with their infant.

Nursing interventions and rationales
1. Allow the parents to see and touch the newborn as soon as possible.
Rationale: The attachment process is facilitated during the critical time after delivery.
2. Provide the patient with information regarding the condition and appearance of the newborn.
Rationale: Keeping the patient informed will lessen her anxiety.
3. Encourage the patient to verbalize her feelings and anxieties related to the newborn.
Rationale: Verbalization of feelings can be therapeutic and serve as a basis for teaching.
4. Involve family members in discussions and inform them of the newborn's condition.

Rationale: Family members can offer support to each other and can help to clarify and reinforce information given to the patient.

Nursing diagnosis
Fear related to excessive bleeding and actual or perceived threat of death
Desired outcome: Patient and family will verbalize feelings about the diagnosis and prognosis.

Nursing interventions and rationales
1. Give accurate information regarding the patient's condition.
Rationale: False reassurance can ultimately lead to mistrust and a failure to accept reality.
2. Be available to the patient and her family for listening, talking, and answering questions.
Rationale: Opportunities to share feelings and concerns with the health care team will lessen anxiety and provide an outlet for expression of emotions.
3. Provide additional supportive persons (relatives, clergy) as necessary.
Rationale: During critical care situations, the nursing staff may not always be available to provide necessary emotional support.

Medical diagnosis
Medical diagnosis for DIC is based on:
• documentation of clinical objective data
• abnormal clotting studies (decreased fibrinogen level and platelet count; increased prothrombin time, partial thromboplastin time, whole blood clotting time, and fibrin degradation products).

Medical treatment
Treatment for DIC includes:
• delivering the fetus and placenta promptly to remove precipitating factors
• replacing intravascular fluid volume with packed red blood cells and crystalloid solutions
• replacing clotting factors, as necessary (Fresh frozen plasma or cryoprecipitate is given to maintain a fibrinogen level above 150 mg/dl. Platelets are indicated if the count is less than 50,000 cells/mm^3 in a patient undergoing surgery.)
• inserting a central venous pressure line or Swan-Ganz pulmonary artery catheter to monitor fluid volume replacement in severe cases (This is done only if the prospective benefit of the procedure outweighs the risk of catheter placement in a patient with inadequate blood-clotting mechanisms.)
• using heparin; may be used in cases involving intrauterine fetal death.

☐ Dystocia

Dystocia refers to difficult labor that is prolonged or more painful because of problems caused by uterine contractions, the fetus, or the bones and tissues of the maternal pelvis. This condition can result in fetal injury or death or in maternal dehydration, infection, or injury.

In dystocia, contractions may be hypotonic (weak) or hypertonic (frequent, painful, and ineffectual). The fetus may be excessively large, malpositioned, or in an abnormal presentation. The maternal pelvis or soft tissues may be too restricted to allow the passage of the fetus.

Patients who experience a prolonged labor, especially if given oxytocin augmentation, are at increased risk for postpartum hemorrhage from uterine atony.

See also "Breech presentation," "Cesarean section," and "Chorioamnionitis" in this section.

Predisposing factors include the following:
• overdistended uterus (from carrying twins or a macrosomatic fetus)
• abnormal positions
• abnormal presentations
• use of analgesics
• chorioamnionitis
• grand multiparity
• advanced maternal age
• postdate pregnancy (fetal head more resistant to molding)
• teenage patient (increased cephalopelvic disproportion)
• fetal anomalies.

Frequently encountered data for dystocia include the following:

Subjective data
• excessive abdominal pain (hypertonic contractions)
• fatigue

Objective data
• abnormal contraction pattern (weak, irregular, or frequent and painful with elevated resting tone of the uterus)
• fetal distress (hypertonic contractions, cephalopelvic disproportion)
• elevated maternal temperature and maternal or fetal tachycardia (chorioamnionitis)
• lack of progress in labor with adequate uterine contractions (cephalopelvic disproportion, abnormal position or presentation, or macrosomia)
• shoulder dystocia (macrosomatic fetus or relative cephalopelvic disproportion)
• ketonuria (inadequate caloric intake because of long labor)
• decreased urine output (dehydration).

Below is a list of nursing diagnoses and interventions frequently associated with dystocia.

Nursing diagnosis
Fluid Volume Deficit related to prolonged labor and restricted fluid intake
Desired outcome: Patient remains well hydrated throughout labor.

Nursing interventions and rationales
1. Administer I.V. fluids, as ordered.
Rationale: I.V. fluids replace fluids lost by the body.
2. Check the patient's lips and mucous membranes for dryness, and assess skin turgor.
Rationale: These are clinical assessments of dehydration.
3. Monitor the patient's fluid intake and output.
Rationale: Such monitoring helps in assessing the fluid balance in the body.

Nursing diagnosis
Pain related to ineffective labor pattern
Desired outcome: Patient is not exhausted and experiences as much comfort as possible.

Nursing interventions and rationales
1. Allow the patient's support person to remain with her as much as possible.
Rationale: The presence of a familiar person reduces fear and relaxes the patient.
2. Coach the patient in breathing techniques and relaxation exercises.
Rationale: These techniques may decrease discomfort. Medication is usually contraindicated (except with hypertonic pattern) to avoid further inhibiting the labor progress.
3. Provide comfort measures, such as back rubs and position changes.
Rationale: These may help the patient to relax and may decrease discomfort.

Nursing diagnosis
High Risk for Infection related to prolonged rupture of the membranes, frequent vaginal examinations, and placement of internal pressure catheter
Desired outcome: Patient develops no infections as a result of labor dystocia.

Nursing interventions and rationales
1. Monitor the patient's temperature and pulse rate every 2 hours.
Rationale: Increased temperature and pulse rate may indicate infection.

2. Cleanse the patient's perineal area before vaginal examinations. (Many institutions use a povidone-iodine solution if the patient is not allergic to iodine.)
Rationale: Cleansing decreases bacteria on skin that can be introduced during examinations.
3. Use sterile examination gloves and good technique during vaginal examinations; use sterile technique during placement of an intrauterine pressure catheter (usually placed by the health care provider).
Rationale: These measures help to minimize the introduction of bacteria.
4. Perform vaginal examinations only when necessary.
Rationale: Progress can be assessed by observing the monitor pattern and the patient's reactions to contractions.

Nursing diagnosis
Altered Placental Tissue Perfusion related to prolonged labor or the use of oxytocic drugs
Desired outcome: Fetus develops no abnormal fetal heart rate patterns during labor.

Nursing interventions and rationales
1. Observe the fetal monitor strip for evidence of distress (see "Fetal monitoring" in Section 3).
Rationale: Decreased variability, or late or variable decelerations, may indicate fetal distress.
2. Observe the color of the amniotic fluid.
Rationale: Meconium staining may indicate fetal distress.
3. Maintain the patient in a lateral position during labor as much as possible.
Rationale: This position increases blood flow to the placenta.
4. Monitor contraction pattern closely for hyperstimulation.
Rationale: Oxytocic drugs used to stimulate labor can produce hypercontractility of the uterus and subsequent fetal distress.

Nursing diagnosis
Fluid Volume Excess related to antidiuretic action of oxytocin
Desired outcome: The patient maintains fluid balance when oxytocin is used.

Nursing interventions and rationales
1. Monitor the patient's fluid intake and output.
Rationale: Monitoring will help in assessing fluid balance in the body.
2. Monitor I.V. infusions closely.
Rationale: Monitoring helps to avoid overhydration with I.V. fluids.

Medical diagnosis

Medical diagnosis for dystocia is based on:
• ultrasound to assess fetal weight, position, and presentation
• intrauterine pressure catheter to evaluate the strength of uterine contractions as well as their frequency and duration
• Freidman labor curve to plot the labor progress
• Calculation of Montivideo units (summation of values at contraction peaks minus value at baseline over a 10-minute period).

Medical treatment

Treatment for dystocia includes:
• adequate maternal hydration and nutrition
• amniotomy if the presenting part is engaged
• fetal monitoring and use of an intrauterine pressure catheter if oxytocin is to be used (see "Fetal monitoring" in Section 3)
• oxytocin augmentation for hypotonic pattern
• sedative or analgesic medication for a hypertonic pattern to stop the abnormal contractions
• cesarean section for cephalopelvic disproportion, breech presentation, and failure to progress in patients with a malpositioned fetus (transverse arrest, occiput posterior) or macrosomatic fetus
• forceps or a vacuum extraction; this is sometimes used to rotate the fetus into a more favorable position or to facilitate delivery when maternal expulsive efforts are inadequate.

☐ Emergency childbirth

Precipitate labor is defined as a labor that lasts less than 3 hours from onset to delivery. Frequently, this occurs because the delivery is not anticipated; consequently, no preparations are made and the health care provider is not in attendance. The nurse must then assume responsibility for managing the patient until the health care provider arrives. With this type of labor, the infant is at risk for hypoxia if contractions have been strong and close together. Rapid propulsion of the fetus through the birth canal can predispose the infant, especially a premature one, to intracranial hemorrhage. Maternal lacerations may occur from rapid descent and delivery of the newborn. The risk of postpartum hemorrhage from uterine atony is increased; uterine rupture and amniotic fluid embolism can also occur.

Predisposing factors include the following:
• grand multiparity
• premature infant
• oxytocin stimulation
• history of rapid labors.

Frequently encountered data for emergency childbirth include the following:

Subjective data
• patient's verbal indication that the delivery is imminent

Objective data
- presenting part crowning on the perineum.

Below is a list of nursing diagnoses and interventions frequently associated with emergency childbirth. (See also "Postpartum hemorrhage" in this section.)

Nursing diagnosis
Fear related to rapid labor progress and the possibility of delivering without medical support
Desired outcome: Patient's fear will be lessened and she will feel reassured by the presence of the nurse.

Nursing interventions and rationales
1. Remain calm and supportive of the patient.
Rationale: Reassuring the patient with a calm, organized approach will enable her to feel confident about her caregivers, even if the primary health care provider is not present.
2. Allow the patient's support person to remain with her.
Rationale: The patient's support person will help to lessen her fear and anxiety.
3. Do not attempt to delay delivery by obstructing the vaginal opening with the patient's legs.
Rationale: Doing so could damage the fetus and increase the patient's discomfort and anxiety.

Medical diagnosis
Not applicable

Medical treatment
Treatment for emergency delivery includes:
- not engaging delivery position of the delivery table if the health care provider is not present
- providing as clean an environment as possible for delivery
- putting on sterile gloves if available
- rupturing the membranes if they are still intact
- supporting the infant's head as it is being delivered
- checking for the cord around the infant's neck
- suctioning the infant's mouth and nares if time permits
- after external rotation, exerting gentle, downward pressure to facilitate delivery of the anterior shoulder
- holding the infant's posterior arm against his body to prevent its tearing the perineum as the body is delivered
- suctioning the infant's mouth and nose thoroughly
- drying the infant and keeping him warm
- if cord ties or clamps are available, clamping and cutting the cord after it stops pulsating
- delivering the placenta (Lengthening of the cord and a slight

gush of blood are signs of placental separation. The patient should be instructed to push; then the placenta should be lifted from the vagina.)
• putting the infant to the patient's breast if bleeding is excessive
• massaging the uterus until it is firm.

☐ Endometritis

An infection of the lining of the uterus after delivery, endometritis is caused by bacteria that usually invade at the placental site and that may spread to involve the entire endometrium. Endometritis may cause peritonitis and pelvic thrombophlebitis or cellulitis.

Predisposing factors include the following:
• prolonged labor
• prolonged rupture of the membranes
• cesarean section
• chorioamnionitis
• maternal hemorrhage
• use of internal monitoring equipment
• anemia
• diabetes
• poor nutritional status
• low socioeconomic status
• obesity
• manual removal of the placenta.

Frequently encountered data for endometritis include the following:

Subjective data
• chilly sensation
• decreased appetite
• headache, backache
• prolonged, severe afterpains
• tender uterus

Objective data
• elevated temperature (greater than 100.4 F [38° C] after the first 24 hours after delivery)
• shaking chills
• increased pulse rate
• large uterus
• foul odor of lochia
• reddish brown lochia
• ileus
• elevated white blood cell count with a left shift (increase in immature forms). Although the white blood cell count is normally elevated postpartum, a left shift usually does not occur unless bacterial infection is present.

Below is a list of nursing diagnoses and interventions frequently associated with endometritis.

Nursing diagnosis
Fluid Volume Deficit related to infectious process
Desired outcome: Fluid volume is maintained or restored.

Nursing interventions and rationales
1. Monitor the patient's fluid intake and output.
Rationale: This will help you assess fluid balance in the body.
2. Encourage the patient to take fluids orally; monitor I.V. fluids.
Rationale: These measures should help to replace fluid volume and to maintain hydration.
3. Administer antibiotics as ordered.
Rationale: Resolution of the infectious process will prevent additional fluid loss.
4. Monitor the patient's vital signs.
Rationale: Decreased blood pressure and increased pulse rate are signs of hypovolemia. Increased temperature is associated with increased fluid loss.

Nursing diagnosis
Pain related to process of infection and spread of infection
Desired outcome: Pain is controlled until infection is resolved.

Nursing interventions and rationales
1. Administer pain medication as ordered, and evaluate the patient's response.
Rationale: Analgesics help minimize patient discomfort.
2. Offer additional comfort measures, such as back rubs and position changes.
Rationale: Comfort measures may relax the patient and lessen discomfort.
3. Observe for signs of increased pain, and report such signs to the health care provider.
Rationale: Increased pain may indicate extension of infection.

Nursing diagnosis
Higk Risk for Altered Parenting related to maternal illness
Desired outcome: Effective maternal-infant bonding occurs.

Nursing interventions and rationales
1. Do not isolate the newborn from the patient.
Rationale: Isolation is usually unnecessary. Be sure to teach the patient proper hand-washing techniques; if possible, keep the newborn in the room with the patient as long as the patient is well enough to assist with care.
2. Allow the patient to see the newborn often if she is too ill to keep the infant with her.

Rationale: Early, frequent interaction will facilitate attachment.
3. Keep the patient informed of her newborn's progress if he is in a special care nursery.
Rationale: Keeping the patient informed helps her to maintain some contact with the newborn; it may prevent her from initiating a grief response if the newborn is progressing well.

Medical diagnosis
Medical diagnosis for endometritis is based on:
• documentation of clinical signs and symptoms
• blood, endometrial, and wound cultures
• catheterized urine specimen to rule out urinary tract infection.

Medical treatment
Treatment for endometritis involves:
• placing the patient in Fowler's position to facilitate drainage of lochia
• administering oxytocic drugs to improve uterine tone
• fluid replacement
• administering I.V. antibiotics to kill both aerobic and anaerobic organisms
• keeping the patient in a private room and ensuring that both the patient and staff observe good hand-washing technique. Patients with infected wounds should be isolated for wound and skin precautions.

☐ Fetal death in utero (FDIU)
FDIU, or fetal demise, is the death of a fetus after the 20th week of gestation and before birth. Disseminated intravascular coagulation (DIC) can develop if the dead fetus is retained in the uterus for 3 to 4 weeks or more because of the release of thromboplastin from the fetal tissues.
   Predisposing factors include the following:
• diabetes
• pregnancy-induced hypertension
• chronic hypertension
• intrauterine growth retardation
• post-date pregnancies
• Rh-sensitized pregnancies
• abruptio placentae.
   Frequently encountered data for fetal death in utero include the following:

Subjective data
• absence of fetal movement

Objective data
• absence of fetal heart tones

• weight loss
• lack of growth or a decrease in fundal height.

Below is a list of nursing diagnoses and interventions frequently associated with fetal death in utero. (See also "Disseminated intravascular coagulation" in this section.)

Nursing diagnosis

Dysfunctional Grieving related to loss of the fetus
Desired outcome: Patient shows progress in dealing with the stages of grief at her own pace.

Nursing interventions and rationales

1. Support the patient's decisions about labor, birth, and the postpartum period, especially if they are known to facilitate the grieving process.
Rationale: Holding the infant after birth, securing mementos (footprints, photographs), and naming the infant can be essential to the normal grieving process.
2. Recognize and identify patient behaviors as normal or abnormal responses to grieving.
Rationale: Anger or hostility can be normal responses and must be accepted by the staff, whereas excessive somatic complaints can be a sign of dysfunctional grieving and indicate that the patient may need professional counseling.
3. Provide the patient with information about the normal patterns of feelings and actions in relation to the stages of grief.
Rationale: Information about the grieving process should help the patient understand that her feelings and actions are a normal, healthy response to her loss. If the patient recognizes which behaviors are outside the normal process, she may accept professional counseling more readily.
4. Refer the patient to the appropriate support groups.
Rationale: These groups provide additional support and follow-up after discharge.

Nursing diagnosis

Fear related to the possibility of future fetal deaths
Desired outcome: Patient verbalizes the cause (if known) of fetal death and the chance of recurrence with subsequent pregnancies.

Nursing interventions and rationales

1. Support and encourage the patient's family to consent to an autopsy if this has been recommended by the health care provider.
Rationale: An autopsy may provide an explanation of the fetal death and of the possibility of recurrence with subsequent pregnancies.
2. Provide an opportunity for the patient and her family to ask questions; answer their questions honestly.

Rationale: Families need open, honest communication to help alleviate fear.

Medical diagnosis

Medical diagnosis for FDIU is based on ultrasound to determine lack of cardiac activity and other characteristics of fetal death.

Medical treatment

Treatment for FDIU includes:
• monitoring clotting studies
• induction of labor.

☐ Heart disease

The incidence of heart disease in pregnancy has declined, probably because of the widespread use of antibiotic therapy for streptococcal infections. In the past, rheumatic heart disease was the most prevalent cardiac problem in pregnancy; recently, an increased incidence of congenital cardiovascular disease has been identified.

More young women with congenital heart defects are having corrective cardiac surgery, thus living longer, marrying, and desiring children. However, these women are also at increased risk for giving birth to children with a similar congenital heart defect (1% to 4% incidence). Some cardiovascular lesions place the woman at high risk for major disability and death (as with Eisenmenger's syndrome and primary pulmonary hypertension), whereas others pose relatively few risks for the mother or her infant.

The New York Heart Association classifies heart disease according to overall functional impairment:

Class I	Asymptomatic
Class II	Symptomatic with heavy exercise
Class III	Symptomatic with light exercise
Class IV	Symptomatic at rest

Many patients progress from a mild classification (I or II) to a more severe form as the hemodynamic stress of pregnancy compromises their cardiac function. Cardiac decompensation places the patient at increased risk for spontaneous abortion, premature labor, fetal death, and maternal death. Newborns tend to be small for their gestational age.

Predisposing factors include the following:
• rheumatic fever
• congenital cardiac defects.

Frequently encountered data for heart disease in pregnancy include the following:

Subjective data
• easy fatigability

- chest discomfort
- dyspnea
- orthopnea
- palpitations
- syncope

Objective data
- peripheral edema
- cough, with or without hemoptysis
- diastolic murmur or systolic murmur greater than Grade 2/6
- cyanosis
- clubbing
- pulmonary crackles
- respiratory distress
- cardiac arrhythmias.

Below is a list of nursing diagnoses and interventions frequently associated with heart disease in pregnancy.

Nursing diagnosis

Activity Intolerance related to increased oxygen requirements during pregnancy
Desired outcome: Patient adjusts to activity restriction and hypoxia does not result.

Nursing interventions and rationales

1. Define an activity level for the patient and monitor her cardiac response; have her report changes in activity tolerance.
Rationale: The patient's activity tolerance often changes during pregnancy. Decreased activity tolerance may signal a deterioration of cardiac function.
2. Teach the patient skills in conserving energy while performing activities of daily living.
Rationale: Conserving energy decreases oxygen consumption while allowing the patient to perform more activities of daily living.
3. Encourage 8 to 10 hours of sleep per night and rest periods during the day in the left lateral position.
Rationale: This decreases oxygen consumption and cardiac work load.
4. Administer iron and folic acid supplements as ordered, and monitor hemoglobin and hematocrit levels when ordered.
Rationale: Anemia increases the cardiac work load.
5. Refer the patient to appropriate social services for help with household responsibilities, as needed.
Rationale: The patient may be unable to resume home care and child care responsibilities because of activity restrictions.

Nursing diagnosis

Altered Placental Tissue Perfusion related to maternal cardiac disease

Desired outcome: The newborn is as appropriate for gestational age at birth as possible in relation to the patient's degree of cardiac compromise.

Nursing interventions and rationales

1. Encourage adequate weight gain (usually not more than 24 pounds) and proper nutrition.
Rationale: Appropriate maternal weight gain and proper maternal nutrition help ensure adequate fetal nutrients without placing additional stress on the patient's cardiovascular system.
2. Instruct the patient to rest frequently in the lateral position.
Rationale: Resting in this position helps increase uterine blood flow.
3. Monitor fundal growth and serial ultrasounds, as ordered.
Rationale: These clinical measures evaluate fetal growth.
4. Perform a nonstress test or contraction stress test beginning at 32 to 34 weeks' gestation, as ordered.
Rationale: Surveillance testing may identify a compromised fetus.

Nursing diagnosis

Decreased Cardiac Output related to increased intravascular fluid volume during pregnancy

Desired outcome: No cardiac complications occur.

Nursing interventions and rationales

1. Promote increased rest periods.
Rationale: Resting decreases cardiac work load.
2. Instruct the patient in following a low-sodium diet, as ordered.
Rationale: Lowered sodium intake prevents fluid retention that increases cardiac work load.
3. Monitor the patient's weight gain; encourage her to avoid excessive weight gain.
Rationale: Excessive weight gain causes increased cardiac work load.
4. Monitor the patient for signs and symptoms of cardiac decompensation.
Rationale: Normal physiologic changes of pregnancy can rapidly precipitate cardiac compromise.
5. Administer medications as ordered; evaluate the patient's response to medication.
Rationale: Many drugs used for cardiac patients, such as diuretics and digoxin, effectively decrease stress on the heart.
6. Observe the patient closely postpartum for fluid volume excess.
Rationale: Normal mobilization of fluids postpartum can cause cardiac decompensation.

Nursing diagnosis

High Risk for Infection related to valvular disease and to invasive procedures in labor and delivery
Desired outcome: No bacterial endocarditis occurs.

Nursing interventions and rationales

1. Instruct the patient in recognizing the signs and symptoms of infection.
Rationale: Early intervention may prevent complications.
2. Instruct the patient regarding medication administration at home; administer medications, as ordered.
Rationale: Prophylactic antibiotics are given to prevent infection.
3. Caution the patient to avoid exposure to infection.
Rationale: Exposure to people with colds and flu places the patient at increased risk for infection.

Nursing diagnosis

Fear related to potential complications for the mother, fetus, and newborn
Desired outcome: Patient is aware of potential risks of pregnancy and expresses her feelings regarding fears and anxieties.

Nursing interventions and rationales

1. Ensure that the patient with known cardiac disease receives preconceptual counseling regarding the risks and potential complications.
Rationale: Patients who choose pregnancy knowing the risks involved may be less anxious.
2. Emphasize to the patient all the normal aspects of the pregnancy.
Rationale: Accentuating the normal aspects may prevent the patient from focusing on how her pregnancy is different from other pregnancies.
3. Allow the patient to verbalize her feelings.
Rationale: Verbalization is therapeutic and serves as a source of information for the nurse for further education and counseling.
4. Explain all procedures and changes in the plan of care to the patient.
Rationale: Because further development of symptoms is common in cardiac diseases, treatment will sometimes change as the pregnancy progresses.
5. Encourage the patient's family to help her cope with her fears during a high-risk pregnancy.
Rationale: Family involvement will improve care and continuity at home.

Medical diagnosis

Medical diagnosis for heart disease is based on:
• ECG
• echocardiogram.

Medical treatment

Treatment for heart disease includes:

• drug therapy, as indicated (diuretics may be necessary)
• putting the patient on a low-sodium diet to prevent fluid retention (usually includes no added salt and restricting foods high in sodium)
• advising the patient to avoid excessive weight gain
• cardiology consultation
• maintaining restricted maternal activity (keeping the patient in the lateral position to increase uterine blood flow)
• administering iron and folic acid to prevent anemia
• administering anticoagulant therapy for patients at risk for thromboembolic events. Note the following:
   — Oral anticoagulants are teratogenic and can only be used during the second trimester.
   — Heparin must be used in the first and third trimesters and is usually the drug of choice throughout pregnancy because it does not cross the placenta.
   — Patients who desire children and who need a valve prosthesis or require a valve replacement should consider a porcine valve because anticoagulant therapy is not required.
• serial sonograms for fetal growth
• nonstress test or contraction stress test beginning at 32 to 34 weeks' gestation
• for patients with history of rheumatic fever and those with rheumatic heart disease, administration of penicillin G benzathine every 4 weeks to prevent streptococcal infection (or administration of sulfadiazine, if the patient is allergic to penicillin)
• for patients with valvular abnormalities and some congenital lesions, administration of antibiotic prophylaxis against endocarditis during labor and delivery
• avoiding the administration of tocolytics (except magnesium sulfate), as they are contraindicated in cardiac patients
• preventing vena cava syndrome in labor
• assisting tissue perfusion with supplemental oxygen
• delivering the newborn with low-outlet forceps to minimize cardiovascular changes during the second stage of labor (epidural anesthesia is often used)
• keeping in mind that the patient is at great risk for postpartum complications as fluid is moved into the cardiovascular system, resulting in circulatory overload (congestive heart failure, pulmonary edema).

☐ HELLP syndrome

This syndrome refers to a complication of pregnancy-induced hypertension involving hemolysis of red blood cells, elevated liver enzyme levels, and a low platelet count. Besides biochemical changes in the patient's liver function, liver rupture, hemorrhage, and death may occur.

For predisposing factors, see "Pregnancy-induced hypertension" in this section.

Frequently encountered data for HELLP syndrome include the following:

Subjective data
- nausea
- moderate to severe epigastric and right upper quadrant pain
- tenderness on liver palpation

Objective data
- vomiting
- hypertension (perhaps not markedly elevated)
- proteinuria
- jaundice
- enlarged liver
- elevated liver enzyme levels, low platelet count, and the presence of schistocytes and burr cells on blood smear.

For a list of nursing diagnoses and interventions frequently associated with HELLP syndrome, see "Disseminated intravascular coagulation" and "Pregnancy-induced hypertension" in this section.

Medical diagnosis
Medical diagnosis for HELLP syndrome is based on:
- documentation of clinical signs and symptoms
- liver function studies
- complete blood count (burr cells and schistocytes on blood smear resulting from hemolysis)
- platelet count
- clotting profile (disseminated intravascular coagulation may develop).

Medical treatment
Treatment for HELLP syndrome includes delivery if liver function changes and thrombocytopenia are prominent.

☐ Hematoma
After delivery, blood may escape into the connective tissues of the reproductive tract to form a hematoma. This potentially life-threatening condition usually follows injury to a blood vessel without laceration of the more superficial tissues; it may occur after spontaneous or operative delivery.

Vulvar hematomas are usually seen externally, diagnosed early, and treated successfully. Hematomas that extend upward and into the broad ligament may escape detection until significant blood loss has occurred.

Predisposing factors for hematomas include operative delivery with forceps.

Frequently encountered data include the following:

Subjective data
• severe pain (abnormal to that experienced postpartum)
• pressure in the perineal area

Objective data
• sensitive tumor seen in the perineal area of varying size covered by discolored skin (vulvar hematoma)
• inability to void
• palpable tumor felt on vaginal examination
• falling hematocrit level
• pallor, tachycardia, and hypotension when significant blood loss occurs.

Below is a list of nursing diagnoses and interventions frequently associated with hematomas (See also "Postpartum hemorrhage" in this section).

Nursing diagnosis
Pain related to pressure of the hematoma on surrounding tissues
Desired outcome: Pain is relieved through resolution of hematoma.

Nursing interventions and rationales
1. Assess the postpartum patient frequently for abnormal pain (especially when forceps delivery occurred).
Rationale: Early diagnosis and intervention may prevent excessive pain and blood loss.
2. Apply ice to the hematoma site, as ordered.
Rationale: Ice promotes comfort and vasoconstricts bleeding vessels.
3. Administer analgesics as ordered, and evaluate the patient's response to medication.
Rationale: Medications may be necessary to control pain until the hematoma resolves or is evacuated.

Nursing diagnosis
Altered Urinary Elimination related to pressure of the hematoma against the urethra
Desired outcome: Patient will have relief of obstruction with complete bladder emptying.

Nursing interventions and rationales
1. Monitor the patient's intake and output carefully.
Rationale: Monitoring makes it possible to assess fluid balance.
2. Check the patient's bladder for distention.
Rationale: The patient may be unaware of the need to void.

3. Employ nursing measures to encourage voiding.
Rationale: Placing warm water over the perineum or the sound of running water may help to stimulate voiding.
4. Catheterize the patient if necessary, as ordered.
Rationale: Patients unable to void may need a catheter until the hematoma is resolved.

Nursing diagnosis
High Risk for Infection related to blood loss and trauma
Desired outcome: Infection does not occur.

Nursing interventions and rationales
1. Monitor the patient for signs and symptoms of infection, including increased temperature, pulse rate, and white blood cell count.
Rationale: Early intervention may prevent complications.
2. Administer antibiotics as ordered, and evaluate the patient's response to medication.
Rationale: Prophylactic antibiotics may be given to prevent infection.
3. Administer perineal care; instruct the patient in self-care measures.
Rationale: Perineal care minimizes the introduction of infection.

Medical diagnosis
Medical diagnosis for hematoma is based on:
• documentation of clinical signs and symptoms
• vaginal examination
• serial hematocrit studies
• ultrasound.

Medical treatment
Treatment for hematoma includes:
• application of ice to decrease edema and to vasoconstrict bleeding vessels
• maintaining fluid and blood replacement
• administration of antibiotics because infection may follow hematoma formation
• catheterization if the patient is unable to void
• incision and evacuation with ligation of the bleeding points.
Note: Hematomas may resolve spontaneously.

☐ Hyperbilirubinemia
Although jaundice caused by hyperbilirubinemia is probably the most common potentially abnormal sign in the immediate neonatal period, only a fraction of affected newborns require intervention. However, when therapy is indicated, it is aimed at preventing kernicterus, which is probably caused by deposition

of bilirubin in brain cells, resulting in permanent neurologic damage.

There are three major types of jaundice associated with hyperbilirubinemia: physiologic, breast-feeding, and pathologic jaundice. *Physiologic jaundice* occurs within 24 to 48 hours after birth, usually as a result of the breakdown of the newborn infant's red blood cells, which increases the load to the liver. Indirect bilirubin levels can rise to 8 to 12 mg/dl by the fourth day after birth, gradually decreasing to less than 1.5 mg/dl by the tenth day. *Breast-feeding jaundice,* thought to be caused by the inhibition of action of glucoronyl transferase by pregnanediol and free fatty acid found in breast milk, usually occurs by the seventh day after birth. Bilirubin levels rise as high as 15 mg/dl or more and last for 2 to 3 weeks before decreasing. *Pathologic jaundice,* which results from conditions increasing bilirubin production, such as hemolytic disease, or reducing its excretion, such as decreased hepatic uptake of bilirubin, most often occurs 24 to 36 hours after birth. Bilirubin levels exceed 12 mg/dl and increase by 5 mg/dl or more daily, indicating a pathologic process.

At any serum bilirubin level, the appearance of jaundice during the first day of life indicates a pathologic process. Diagnostic evaluation is also indicated when serum levels are over 12 mg/dl in term newborns (15 mg/dl preterm), levels rise more than 5 mg/dl in 24 hours, or jaundice persists beyond 7 days (10 to 14 days preterm).

Predisposing factors for hyperbilirubinemia include the following:
• Rh or ABO maternal-fetal incompatibility
• polycythemia
• cephalohematoma
• drug toxicity
• sepsis
• maternal diabetes
• premature birth
• certain maternal medications
• asphyxia
• cold stress.

Frequently encountered data for hyperbilirubinemia include the following:

Subjective data
Not applicable

Objective data
• jaundice
• elevated serum bilirubin levels
• enlarged liver
• poor muscle tone
• lethargy
• poor sucking reflex.

Below is a nursing diagnosis and related interventions frequently associated with hyperbilirubinemia.

Nursing diagnosis
High Risk for Injury: Kernicterus related to hyperbilirubinemia
Desired outcome: Serum bilirubin levels remain below 20 mg/dl.

Nursing interventions and rationales
1. Observe the newborn every 4 hours for level of jaundice.
Rationale: Clinical observation may detect newborns who are developing hyperbilirubinemia.
2. Keep the newborn well hydrated.
Rationale: Hydration helps maintain blood volume and encourages excretion of bilirubin in the urine.
3. Facilitate early, frequent breast-feeding to hasten passage of meconium.
Rationale: Bilirubin can be reabsorbed into the circulation from the meconium in the newborn's intestines.
4. Report any signs of jaundice in the first 24 hours and any abnormal signs and symptoms to the health care provider.
Rationale: Early intervention will prevent bilirubin levels from escalating to dangerous levels.
5. Monitor the newborn closely during phototherapy (see "Phototherapy" in Section 3).
Rationale: Injury from treatment, such as eye damage, dehyration, or sensory deprivation, can occur.

Medical diagnosis
Medical diagnosis for hyperbilirubinemia is based on:
• documentation of clinical signs and symptoms
• serum bilirubin levels.

Medical treatment
Treatment includes:
• adequate hydration
• phototherapy (see "Phototherapy" in Section 3)
• exchange transfusion.
New research has revealed that the newborn can tolerate a higher level of bilirubin without injury. Therefore, treatment may be initiated at somewhat higher levels.

☐ Hyperemesis gravidarum
Also known as pernicious nausea and vomiting of pregnancy, hyperemesis gravidarum is intractable nausea and vomiting that persists beyond the first trimester with resulting disturbances in nutrition, electrolytes, and fluid balance.
Predisposing factors include the following:
• history of hyperemesis gravidarum

• multiple gestations
• hydatidiform mole
• difficulty in adapting to the psychological adjustment of pregnancy and the role of mothering.
  Frequently encountered data for hyperemesis gravidarum include the following:

Subjective data
• nausea (most pronounced on arising; however, it may also occur at other times during the day)
• thirst
• lethargy

Objective data
• persistent vomiting
• weight loss
• electrolyte disturbances (decreased potassium, sodium, and chloride levels)
• ketonuria
• oliguria
• hypotension
• decreased skin turgor, dry skin, and dry mucous membranes
• constipation
• high hematocrit level
• fever
• tachycardia.
  Below is a list of nursing diagnoses and interventions frequently associated with hyperemesis gravidarum.

Nursing diagnosis
Altered Nutrition: Less Than Body Requirements related to inability to retain food
Desired outcome: Patient will be able to retain food in sufficient amounts to sustain herself and the developing fetus during pregnancy.

Nursing interventions and rationales
1. Instruct the patient to restrict oral intake, as ordered, until vomiting subsides.
Rationale: The sight and smell of food can trigger vomiting, resulting in further depletion of fluid and electrolytes.
2. Monitor I.V. therapy used to correct hypovolemia, restore electrolyte balance, and provide nutrition for mother and fetus.
Rationale: Restoration of fluid and electrolyte balance often resolves the process of recurrent vomiting. Total parenteral nutrition is sometimes necessary in severe, persistent cases.
3. Record the patient's weight daily.
Rationale: A daily weight record is important in monitoring the progress of therapy.
4. Record the patient's intake and output and calorie count.

Rationale: These records make it possible to evaluate fluid balance and serve as a basis for I.V. therapy. Calorie count approximates actual nutrient intake.

5. Check the patient's urine for ketones.

Rationale: Ketones in the urine indicate maternal fat consumption for energy because of inadequate caloric intake.

6. Administer antiemetics as ordered.

Rationale: Phenothiazines are sometimes ordered to control vomiting.

7. Begin the patient on a dry diet, as ordered, alternating liquids and solids in small quantities.

Rationale: Taking solids and liquids at alternate times decreases nausea and vomiting.

8. Advance the patient's diet slowly as she becomes more tolerant.

Rationale: Gradual reintroduction of foods improves the success of therapy.

9. Monitor fetal heart tones and fetal activity.

Rationale: Fetal heart tones within normal limits and an active fetus are indications of fetal well-being.

10. Assess fundal height weekly.

Rationale: Increasing fundal height indicates fetal growth.

Nursing diagnosis

Fluid Volume Deficit related to excessive vomiting
Desired outcome: Fluid balance will be restored and maintained during pregnancy.

Nursing interventions and rationales

1. Monitor the patient's serum electrolyte levels, as ordered.

Rationale: Monitoring enables evaluation of the therapy's effectiveness and serves as a basis for replacement guidelines.

2. Monitor I.V. therapy, as ordered.

Rationale: I.V. therapy restores fluid volume and allows for electrolyte replacement.

3. Monitor the patient's intake and output.

Rationale: Such monitoring serves as a guide for fluid replacement. Urine output greater than 30 ml/hour indicates normal renal perfusion.

4. Assess the patient's skin texture and turgor.

Rationale: Dry skin and decreased skin turgor are signs of dehydration.

5. Monitor the patient's vital signs.

Rationale: Decreased blood pressure and increased pulse rate and temperature are signs of dehydration and hypovolemia.

Nursing diagnosis

Ineffective Individual Coping related to the psychological demands of pregnancy and approaching motherhood

Desired outcome: Patient adapts to the psychological demands of pregnancy and approaching motherhood.

Nursing interventions and rationales
1. Encourage the patient to verbalize her feelings regarding the pregnancy.
Rationale: Verbalization of feelings can be therapeutic and serves as a basis for intervention.
2. Restrict visitors, as necessary, to provide a relaxed, calm atmosphere.
Rationale: Minimizing sources of stress will promote needed rest and sleep.
3. Initiate social service assistance to help coordinate care of children at home and to attend to the patient's economic needs.
Rationale: Concern for dependent children and loss of income can impede recovery.
4. Refer the patient for professional psychological intervention, as needed.
Rationale: Psychological evaluation is often helpful in providing emotional and psychological support.

Medical diagnosis
Medical diagnosis for hyperemesis gravidarum is based on:
• documentation of clinical signs and symptoms
• serum electrolyte levels
• urinalysis
• hemoglobin and hematocrit levels.

Medical treatment
Treatment for hyperemesis gravidarum includes:
• hospitalization
• I.V. fluids and electrolyte replacement
• Total parenteral nutrition, as needed
• administration of antiemetics
• serial sonograms to assess fetal growth
• psychiatric consultation, as needed.

☐ Hypoglycemia (neonatal)
During the first 72 hours of life, term newborns are diagnosed as hypoglycemic if plasma glucose levels are less than 30 mg/dl. With low-birth-weight newborns, the lower limit of normal for plasma glucose levels during the first 72 hours of life is 20 mg/dl.

Central nervous system (CNS) dysfunction occurs frequently in untreated symptomatic infants. Prompt recognition and treatment of symptomatic and asymptomatic infants is necessary to minimize neurologic damage; untreated hypoglycemia can cause death.

Predisposing factors include the following:
- diabetic mother
- intrauterine growth retardation
- hypothermia
- asphyxia
- sepsis
- erythroblastosis fetalis
- CNS hemorrhage or malformation
- maternal administration of large amounts of dextrose solution just before delivery.

Frequently encountered data for hypoglycemia include the following:

Subjective data
Not applicable

Objective data
- apnea
- cyanosis
- hypothermia
- rapid, irregular respirations
- tachypnea
- tremors
- lethargy
- pallor
- sweating
- upward rolling of the eyes
- weak cry
- poor feeding
- seizures
- coma.

Below is a nursing diagnosis with appropriate nursing interventions and rationales frequently associated with hypoglycemia.

Nursing diagnosis
High Risk for Injury related to hypoglycemia
Desired outcome: Hypoglycemia is identified and treated so that neurologic damage does not occur.

Nursing interventions and rationales
1. Promote thermoregulation.
Rationale: Glucose is used for energy by the newborn in an attempt to raise body temperature.
2. Check the infant's blood glucose concentration after delivery, as ordered.
Rationale: Hypoglycemia can occur in the absence of predisposing factors.
3. Closely observe the newborn at risk, and perform frequent blood glucose determinations.

Rationale: Newborns predisposed to developing hypoglycemia need to be monitored more intensely.

4. Promote early feedings and prompt treatment of low blood glucose concentration.

Rationale: Prevention of extremely low blood glucose levels will prevent neurologic damage.

Medical diagnosis

Medical diagnosis for hypoglycemia is based on:
• checking blood glucose levels (heel stick)
• venipuncture for blood glucose levels to confirm the results obtained by heel stick.

Medical treatment

Treatment for hypoglycemia includes:
• administering dextrose 10% in water by mouth or gavage
• I.V. administration of a concentrated glucose solution if infant is unable to tolerate oral feedings or if blood glucose level is extremely low.

☐ Intrauterine growth retardation (IUGR)

Newborns whose birth weight, for reasons other than heredity, falls below the 10th percentile expected for their gestational age are termed growth-retarded. Growth-retarded newborns have an increased risk of perinatal morbidity and mortality and are estimated to account for 25% of the entire perinatal mortality.

Predisposing factors include the following:
• low socioeconomic status
• pregnancy-induced hypertension
• chronic hypertension
• chronic renal disease
• diabetes (with vascular disease)
• malnutrition
• smoking
• drug addiction
• alcoholism
• multiple gestation
• congenital or chromosomal anomaly
• chronic intrauterine infection
• placental insufficiency.

Frequently encountered data for intrauterine growth retardation include the following:

Subjective data

None

Objective data

Prenatal
• lagging fundal height growth

• weight loss or poor weight gain
• failure of normal growth on ultrasound
• oligohydramnios
• meconium-stained amniotic fluid

Newborn
• normal skull but reduced dimensions of the rest of the body, making the skull look large
• decreased or absent vernix
• lack of subcutaneous fat
• loose, dry skin
• wide-eyed look
• sunken abdomen (scaphoid)
• thin, yellowish, dry umbilical cord
• sparse scalp hair
• wide skull sutures (inadequate bone growth)
• hypoglycemia.

Below is a nursing diagnosis with appropriate interventions and rationales frequently associated with intrauterine growth retardation. (See also "Hypoglycemia" and "Meconium aspiration syndrome" in this section.)

Nursing diagnosis
High Risk for Injury related to placental insufficiency or postnatal complications in intrauterine growth retardation
Desired outcome: Infant has no permanent damage from complications associated with intrauterine growth retardation.

Nursing interventions and rationales
1. Use an internal fetal monitor during labor. Observe closely for signs of fetal distress.
Rationale: An internal fetal monitor is a more clinically accurate method of detecting fetal distress, which is increased by placental insufficiency and by cord compression associated with decreased amniotic fluid.
2. Encourage the patient to use the lateral position.
Rationale: This position promotes uterine perfusion.
3. Prepare for delivery of a compromised infant. If meconium is present, prepare for proper suctioning.
Rationale: Immediate resuscitation may be necessary. Direct visualization of the cords and suctioning are necessary to prevent meconium aspiration syndrome.
4. Perform frequent blood glucose determinations on the newborn after delivery.
Rationale: Hypoglycemia is a common result of deficient fat stores.
5. Protect the newborn from hypothermia.
Rationale: Lack of subcutaneous fat makes maintenance of body temperature difficult.

Medical diagnosis

Medical diagnosis for IUGR is based on:
• serial ultrasound examinations (at least 3 weeks apart) that demonstrate lack of adequate growth
• oligohydramnios seen on ultrasound
• documentation of clinical signs and symptoms
• evaluating the fetus for chromosomal anomalies. (The health care provider may elect to order such evaluation because infants with chromosomal anomalies are frequently growth-retarded. If the defect is found to be incompatible with life, the patient can be spared an unnecessary cesarean section.)

Medical treatment

Treatment for IUGR includes:
• control of causative factors (cessation of smoking, controlling hypertension, improving nutrition)
• promoting additional rest periods in left lateral position, which increases uteroplacental blood flow
• performing nonstress tests or contraction stress tests
• delivery if fetal surveillance testing indicates fetal jeopardy
• symptomatic treatment after delivery
• chromosomal studies or infectious disease studies to determine the cause(s) of failure to grow.

☐ Large for gestational age (LGA)

A newborn who is plotted above the 90th percentile on the intra-uterine growth curve is large for gestational age. Birth weights over 8 lb, 13 oz (4,000 g) may reflect the genetic predisposition of the fetus or may be associated with maternal diabetes or excessive weight gain in pregnancy. The mortality for large infants born at or near term is higher than for average-sized infants. Shoulder dystocia has been reported in 10% of LGA infants; other birth trauma, in as many as 15% of LGA infants.

Predisposing factors include the following:
• diabetic mother
• post-date pregnancies
• maternal obesity
• excessive maternal weight gain
• multiparity.

Frequently encountered data for LGA include the following:

Subjective data

None

Objective data

Prenatal
• fundal height greater than gestational age
• excessive maternal weight gain
• macrosomia on ultrasound
• dysfunctional labor

Newborn
- birth weight greater than 8 lb 13 oz (4,000 g)
- hypoglycemia, hypocalcemia, hyperbilirubinemia
- respiratory distress syndrome.

For nursing diagnoses and interventions frequently associated with LGA newborns, see "Birth trauma," "Diabetes mellitus," "Hyperbilirubinemia," "Hypoglycemia," and "Respiratory distress syndrome" in this section.

Medical diagnosis
Medical diagnosis for LGA newborns is based on:
- documentation of clinical signs and symptoms
- ultrasound for estimated fetal weight.

Medical treatment
Treatment for LGA newborns includes:
Maternal
- fostering good diabetic control to minimize hyperglycemia
- counseling to control maternal weight gain
- cesarean section for dysfunctional labor with suspected macrosomia to minimize chances of shoulder dystocia

Newborn
- observing for birth trauma and treating accordingly
- performing frequent blood glucose determinations
- observing for signs and symptoms of hypocalcemia
- monitoring bilirubin levels
- monitoring for respiratory distress syndrome.

☐ Mastitis
Mastitis is an inflammation of the breast caused by *Staphylococcus aureus* or hemolytic streptococci. Trauma to the nipples during nursing provides a portal of entry for the organisms, and breast milk provides an excellent medium for bacterial growth. Mastitis most commonly occurs during the 3rd or 4th week postpartum and can progress to abscess formation in severe cases.

Predisposing factors include the following:
- sore, cracked nipples
- improper emptying of the breasts.

Frequently encountered data for mastitis include the following:

Subjective data
- pain
- tenderness to the touch
- malaise
- chills

Objective data
- engorgement
- erythema of the breast

- palpable firm mass in the breast
- cracked nipples
- increased temperature and pulse rate
- increased white blood cell count
- axillary adenopathy.

Below is a list of nursing diagnoses and interventions frequently associated with mastitis.

Nursing diagnosis
Pain related to infectious process
Desired outcome: Pain is relieved or controlled.

Nursing interventions and rationales
1. Apply good breast support.
Rationale: This will support inflamed tissues and prevent tension and pulling.
2. Apply heat, as ordered.
Rationale: Heat increases blood flow to the affected area, thus helping in the resolution of the infectious process.
3. Administer analgesics as ordered, and monitor the patient's response to medication.
Rationale: By depressing the central nervous system, analgesics decrease pain.
4. Encourage frequent breast-feeding.
Rationale: Emptying the breasts decreases engorgement; this helps to eliminate pain.

Nursing diagnosis
High Risk for Altered Parenting related to anxiety over infection and possible discontinuation of breast-feeding
Desired outcome: Anxiety is minimized so as not to interfere with maternal-infant attachment.

Nursing interventions and rationales
1. Encourage the patient to verbalize her feelings about the infection and about changes in feeding plans.
Rationale: The patient may feel guilty if she decides to stop breast-feeding. Her perceptions of the infection and of its effects provide a basis for teaching.
2. Encourage frequent contact with the infant if the patient is too ill to provide total care.
Rationale: Frequent contact reinforces maternal-infant ties.
3. Reassure the patient regarding a successful resolution of the infection.
Rationale: Mastitis usually resolves without further complications.
4. Reassure the patient regarding the infant's ability to adjust to the changes brought about by the infection.
Rationale: Infants usually adjust well to formula feeding.

Medical diagnosis

Medical diagnosis for mastitis is based on:
• documentation of clinical signs and symptoms
• bacterial cultures of the breast milk.

Medical treatment

Treatment for mastitis includes:
• administering antibiotics
• local applications of heat (or cold)
• keeping the breasts empty
• providing good breast support
• continuing with breast-feeding during treatment; continued nursing helps empty the breasts, thus helping resolve the infection. Some patients, however, elect to stop nursing.
• incision and drainage when abscess formation occurs.

☐ Meconium aspiration syndrome (MAS)

The passage of meconium in utero is caused by reflex relaxation of the anal sphincter and accelerated intestinal peristalsis in response to fetal hypoxia. Reflex gasping by the fetus tends to draw the meconium into the tracheobronchial tree. Meconium acts as a foreign body in the lung, blocking the flow of air in the alveoli while producing a chemical pneumonia.

Careful suctioning before delivery (and before initiation of respirations) as well as intubation and deep suctioning after delivery can minimize the incidence of MAS.

Predisposing factors include the following:
• fetal distress
• improper suctioning at delivery.

Frequently encountered data for meconium aspiration syndrome include the following:

Subjective data

Not applicable

Objective data

• difficulty establishing respirations
• crackles heard during lung auscultation
• grunting, tachypnea, retractions, flaring of nares.

Below is a nursing diagnosis with corresponding interventions and rationales frequently associated with MAS.

Nursing diagnosis

Impaired Gas Exchange related to alveolar blockage and chemical pneumonia
Desired outcome: Adequate oxygenation to tissues is maintained.

Nursing interventions and rationales

1. Perform careful and thorough suctioning after delivery of the newborn.

Rationale: Removal of as much of the meconium as possible will minimize the degree of airway obstruction.
2. Monitor the newborn at risk for symptoms.
Rationale: Prompt recognition and treatment minimizes complications.
3. Initiate ventilatory support as ordered when the newborn becomes symptomatic.
Rationale: Such support should maintain adequate tissue oxygenation.

Medical diagnosis
Medical diagnosis for MAS is based on:
• documentation of clinical signs and symptoms
• chest X-ray.

Medical treatment
Treatment consists of the following:
• prevention through proper suctioning
• mechanical ventilation
• supportive care
• extracorporeal membrane oxygenation (ECMO).

☐ Multiple gestation
Multiple gestations can be caused by double ovulation (fraternal, or dizygotic) or a splitting of the fertilized egg (identical, or monozygotic). The incidence of multiple gestations has increased as a result of the increased use of fertility drugs. Common complications with multiple gestations include spontaneous abortion, anemia, congenital anomalies, hyperemesis gravidarum, intrauterine growth retardation, pregnancy-induced hypertension, polyhydramnios, postpartum hemorrhage, premature rupture of the membranes, and preterm labor and delivery.
    Predisposing factors include the following:
• family history of multiple births
• use of fertility drugs
• maternal age between 35 and 39
• increased parity
• recent use of oral contraceptives
• black race (incidence among Nigerian Blacks is 1:25).
    Frequently encountered data for multiple gestation include the following:

Subjective data
• excessive fetal activity

Objective data
• uterus large for gestational age
• palpation of three or four large parts in the uterus
• excessive morning sickness
• auscultation of more than one fetal heart

- pregnancy-induced hypertension
- anemia
- preterm labor
- hemorrhoids
- varicosities
- excessive dependent edema
- excessive weight gain.

Below is a nursing diagnosis with corresponding interventions and rationales frequently associated with multiple gestation. (See also "Anemia," "Cesarean section," "Hyperemesis gravidarum," "Intrauterine growth retardation," "Postpartum hemorrhage," "Pregnancy-induced hypertension," "Preterm birth," and "Preterm labor" in this section.)

Nursing diagnosis
Ineffective Family Coping: Compromised, related to diagnosis of multiple gestation and the implications for altered lifestyle
Desired outcome: Family members express their feelings about having more than one child and make plans for their needs.

Nursing interventions and rationales
1. Allow the family time to verbalize their feelings.
Rationale: Verbalization is therapeutic and serves as a guide for teaching and referral.
2. Consult social service organizations, if necessary.
Rationale: Such pregnancies are considered high-risk; infants may need intensive care after delivery. The family may qualify for financial or medical care assistance.
3. Refer the patient to appropriate support groups after delivery.
Rationale: The National Organization of Mothers of Twins clubs have chapters in many cities and can be of help to such families. Neonatal intensive care units often have support groups if the infants require specialized care as a result of premature delivery.

Medical diagnosis
Medical diagnosis for multiple gestation is based on ultrasound.

Medical treatment
Treatment for multiple gestation includes:
- serial ultrasound for fetal growth
- close monitoring for cervical changes
- treating preterm labor promptly if it occurs
- additional bed rest with the patient in the lateral position
- fetal surveillance using the nonstress test (contraction stress test is contraindicated because of the risk of preterm labor)
- supplemental iron and vitamins
- delivery by cesarean section for abnormal presentations
- oxytocic drugs after delivery to prevent postpartum hemorrhage caused by uterine overdistention.

☐ Perinatal infection

The fetus and newborn can be exposed to numerous infectious agents during pregnancy, delivery, and the neonatal period. Maternal antepartal infections, such as cytomegalovirus, syphilis, rubella, and toxoplasmosis may cause congenital infection. Women harboring such organisms as beta-hemolytic streptococci, *Chlamydia*, HIV, hepatitis B, human papillomavirus (HPV), or gonorrhea during labor may infect their newborns as they pass through the birth canal. (For more information, see *Perinatal infections*, pages 122 and 123, and "Acquired immunodeficiency syndrome" in this section.)

Nursing diagnosis

High Risk for Infection related to maternal disease
Desired outcome: Patient is properly identified, screened, and treated as necessary.

Nursing interventions and rationales

1. Teach the patient how to prevent infection; for example, avoiding handling or changing cat litter, using gloves when gardening, avoiding children with rashes, and using condoms during vaginal intercourse.
Rationale: Many infections can be prevented through patient education.
2. Obtain a thorough health history and results of a thorough physical examination.
Rationale: Such information aids in identifying previous or current infections or exposure.
3. Perform appropriate laboratory tests, as ordered, during pregnancy.
Rationale: Laboratory tests can help identify active infection so that treatment can be implemented.
4. Provide appropriate treatments as ordered.
Rationale: Rubella vaccine can protect subsequent pregnancies; penicillin during labor may protect the infant from Group B streptococcus; neonatal eye prophylaxis protects against *Chlamydia* and gonorrhea; hepatitis B vaccine prevents both maternal and neonatal infection.

Nursing diagnosis

Self-Esteem Disturbance related to awareness of impact of the disease on the patient's own lifestyle and on her relationship with others
Desired outcome: The patient verbalizes feelings of improved self-esteem and methods of coping with existing problems.

Nursing interventions and rationales

1. Provide an opportunity for the patient to discuss feelings, ask questions, and express concerns.

PERINATAL INFECTIONS

Numerous infections can cause problems for the mother and fetus during pregnancy and for the neonate after delivery. The chart below lists the major perinatal infections and the predisposing factors associated with each. Maternal and fetal or neonatal assessment findings also are listed. It is essential for nurses to keep this information in mind when caring for the pregnant patient and her fetus.

Infection	Predisposing Factors	Maternal Assessment Findings	Fetal or Neonatal Assessment Findings
Chlamydia	• Young women having intercourse with a new partner within the preceding 2 months • History of chlamydial infection or other sexually transmitted disease (STD) • Current infection with other STD • Use of nonbarrier contraceptives • Women whose sexual partners have nongonococcal urethritis	• Increased discharge and itching • Friable cervix • Low-grade fever • Abdominal pain, right upper quadrant • Bleeding between periods • Dysuria • Mucopurulent cervicitis	• Conjunctivitis (watery eye discharge, conjunctival hyperemia, mucopurulent discharges) • Pneumonia (barking cough, lung congestion, tachypnea, weight loss, absence of fever)
Gonorrhea	• Presence of other STD • Sexual partner with gonorrhea	• Increased vaginal discharge, purulent • Abdominal pain • Dysuria, frequency • Fever • Arthritis-like symptoms	• Conjunctivitis
Hepatitis B	• Intravenous drug use • Recipients of blood transfusions • Recipients of hemodialysis • Frequent contact with blood and blood products	• Malaise • Headache • Anorexia, nausea • Pruritus • Hepatosplenomegaly • Jaundice • Cervical lymphadenopathy • Abnormal liver function tests	• None at birth but infant is at high risk to develop Hepatitis B infection if not treated with Hepatitis B vaccine or Hepatitis B immune globulin
Group B streptococcus	• Maternal vaginal colonization • Prematurity • Low birth weight • Premature rupture of membranes • Intrapartum maternal fever	*Antepartal* (many patients are asymptomatic) • Premature rupture of membranes *Postpartal* • Elevated temperature • Tachycardia • Abdominal distention • Symptoms of endometritis • Premature labor	*Early onset* • Respiratory distress • Apnea • Pulmonary infiltrates on chest x-ray • Septic shock • Jaundice *Late onset* • Irritability, lethargy • Apnea • Poor feeding • Fever • Symptoms of meningitis

Infection	Predisposing Factors	Maternal Assessment Findings	Fetal or Neonatal Assessment Findings
Herpes	• Sexual partner with herpes • Oral herpes lesions • History of herpes	• Pain • Clusters of vesicles or crusted lesions on perineum • Lymphadenopathy and fever with initial outbreak	• Skin lesions • Hepatosplenomegaly • Petechiae • Anemia • Irritability • Seizures • Poor muscle tone • Jaundice • Disseminated intravascular coagulation
Human papilloma-virus (HPV)	• Sexual contact with HPV infected individual	• Visible warts on perineal area • Cervical cytology suggestive of HPV changes	• None at birth but may develop laryngeal papillomatosis
Rubella	• Nonimmune maternal status • Maternal infection during pregnancy	• Skin rash	• Skin lesions • Cataracts • Heart defects • Anemia • Jaundice • Pneumonitis
Syphilis	• Sexual partner with syphilis • Maternal infection during pregnancy	• Painless genital lesions • Skin rash	• Hepatosplenomegaly • Anemia • Flat, moist skin lesions
Cytomega-lovirus (CMV)	• Low income status • Young, primiparous, unmarried, or poorly educated mother • Past or current CMV infection	• Malaise • Myalgia • Chills • Fever • Leukocytosis	• Jaundice • Anemia • Growth retardation • Microcephaly • Seizures
Toxoplas-mosis	• Maternal contact with cat feces, soil, or undercooked meat • Maternal infection during gestation	• Malaise • Sore throat • Fatigue • Lymphadenopathy • Fever	• Hepatosplenomegaly • Jaundice • Petechiae • Anemia • Thrombocytopenia • Cataracts • Seizures • Hydrocephaly • Hypothermia • Chorioretinitis • Intracranial calcifications

Rationale: Ventilation of feelings is therapeutic and serves as a basis for teaching.

2. Include the patient's partner in discussion sessions.
Rationale: It may be helpful for the patient's partner to discuss the particular infection with a nurse or other health care professional.

3. Refer the patient to appropriate professional counseling or support groups.
Rationale: The patient may need additional support after discharge.

Nursing diagnosis

Knowledge Deficit related to transmission of infection and the infection's effect on pregnancy and on the fetus and newborn
Desired outcome: The patient verbalizes an understanding of the disease and of its impact on the pregnancy.

Nursing interventions and rationales

1. Assess the patient's level of knowledge.
Rationale: This assessment can serve as a basis for the teaching plan.

2. Provide the patient with information, as required.
Rationale: The patient needs information to understand the disease process.

3. Review the treatment plan and explain which symptoms the patient should report to the health care professional.
Rationale: The patient's involvement in the monitoring of the infection may increase compliance.

Medical diagnosis

Medical diagnosis for perinatal infections is based on specific findings for each infection:

Toxoplasmosis
• elevated IgM serum antibody levels
• intracranial calcifications on skull X-ray
• Sabin-Feldman dye test

Rubella
• elevated IgM levels
• pharyngeal cultures

Syphilis
• positive Venereal Disease Research Laboratory (VDRL) test
• positive fluorescent treponemal antibody test

Cytomegalovirus (CMV)
• elevated IgM levels
• cultures for CMV
• skull x-ray for calcifications

Herpes
• culture of lesions

Gonorrhea
• positive culture

Chlamydia
• positive culture

HPV
• visible warts
• cervical cytology suggestive of HPV infection

Hepatitis B
• clinical signs and symptoms
• positive hepatitis B surface antigen/negative hepatitis B surface antibody.

Medical treatment
Treatment for perinatal infections centers primarily around pharmacologic therapy. Some examples include:

Toxoplasmosis
• pyrimethamine, sulfonamides, and folic acid supplements

Chlamydia
• tetracycline for nonpregnant patients; erythromycin for pregnant patients and infants

HPV
• Trichloroacetic acid for small external warts

Syphilis
• penicillin for maternal or congenital syphilis

Herpes
• cesarean section if lesions are present at term
• analgesics and topical anesthetics
• antiviral agents for neonatal herpes

Group B Streptococcus
• antibiotics, ventilatory assistance and fluid and electrolyte therapy for the infant
• penicillin intrapartally for maternal infection

Gonorrhea
• ceftriaxone
• concomitant treatment for *Chlamydia* with erythromycin

Hepatitis B
• Hepatitis B immune globulin for maternal exposure
• Hepatitis B immune globulin for infants born to chronic carriers within 12 hours of birth
• Hepatitis B vaccine started within 48 hours of birth
• no breast-feeding for carriers.

☐ Placenta previa

Placenta previa is the implantation of the placenta near or over the internal os of the cervix. This condition can occur in varying degrees: total or complete placenta previa occurs when the placenta entirely covers the internal os; partial placenta previa occurs when the placenta covers only part of the internal os; marginal placenta previa, or a low-lying placenta, refers to one that is implanted low in the uterus but does not cover the internal os. (See *Complete placenta previa*.)

Placenta previa is the most common cause of bleeding during the last half of pregnancy. The first bleeding episode is rarely fatal. Bleeding usually occurs in the latter half of pregnancy when development of the lower uterine segment loosens the attachment of the placenta to the uterine wall.

Postpartum hemorrhage is increased in patients with this condition because of the inability of the lower uterine segment to contract well after the delivery of the placenta. Maternal mortality is less than 1%; perinatal mortality may be as high as 10% to 15%.

Predisposing factors include the following:
• twins
• erythroblastosis fetalis
• previous cesarean section
• previous placenta previa
• recent dilatation and curettage
• history of myomectomy
• history of endometritis
• maternal age over 35
• multiparity.

Frequently encountered data for placenta previa include the following:

Subjective data
Usually not applicable

Objective data
• painless vaginal bleeding (usually after the 28th week of gestation)
• abnormal fetal position (breech or transverse lie)
• high presenting part
• uterine contractions.

Below is a list of nursing diagnoses and interventions frequently associated with placenta previa.

Nursing diagnosis
Fluid Volume Deficit related to bleeding
Desired outcome: Patient will maintain adequate tissue perfusion.

Nursing interventions and rationales
1. Assess vaginal bleeding and vital signs frequently. (The time interval depends on the patient's status.)

COMPLETE PLACENTA PREVIA

In placenta previa, the placenta is implanted in the lower uterine segment. Because nutrients aren't as abundant in the lower uterus as in the fundus, the placenta migrates to find better nourishment, becoming larger and thinner. As a result, it encroaches on or covers the internal cervical os. The three types of placenta previa are *marginal* (part of the placenta is attached to the lower uterine segment, with the edge at the margin of the internal cervical os), *partial* (the placenta partially covers the internal os), and *complete* or *total* (the placenta entirely covers the internal os, as illustrated).

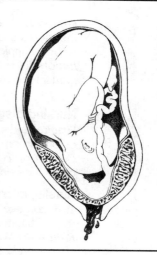

Rationale: Increased bleeding, decreased blood pressure, or increased pulse rate suggests hypovolemia.

2. Encourage the patient to maintain bed rest or limited activity.
Rationale: Activity may precipitate or increase bleeding.

3. Monitor I.V. fluids to help restore circulating fluid volume. (An 18G needle should be used.)
Rationale: I.V. fluids help maintain circulatory volume and provide a route for rapid administration of blood and fluids, if necessary.

4. Administer iron supplements as prescribed.
Rationale: Iron is a necessary component of hemoglobin that enables the red blood cells to carry oxygen.

5. Administer blood as ordered, and observe the patient for reactions.
Rationale: Blood transfusions may be necessary to restore blood volume and maintain tissue perfusion.

Nursing diagnosis

Altered Placental Tissue Perfusion related to inadequate oxygenation
Desired outcome: Adequate placental perfusion and fetal oxygenation will be maintained.

Nursing interventions and rationales

1. Monitor fetal heart rate, fetal activity, and results of fetal surveillance tests when ordered.
Rationale: Alterations in placental perfusion decreases fetal oxygenation, causing decreased activity and abnormal fetal heart rate response.

2. Encourage the patient to maintain a lateral position in bed.

Rationale: The lateral position provides optimum circulation to the uterus and placenta.

3. Give supplemental oxygen as ordered.

Rationale: Supplemental oxygen increases the amount of oxygen available to the fetus.

Nursing diagnosis

Fear related to possible negative effect of bleeding on the patient or on the pregnancy outcome

Desired outcome: Patient will verbalize feelings related to concerns for personal and fetal well-being.

Nursing interventions and rationales

1. Encourage the patient to verbalize anxieties and fears related to the diagnosis and prognosis.

Rationale: Verbalization of feelings can be therapeutic; it may also provide the nurse with insight into the patient's perceptions of the diagnosis and serve as a basis for teaching.

2. Allow the patient to listen to fetal heart tones (if they are present and within normal limits).

Rationale: Listening to the fetal heart tones may provide reassurance of fetal well-being.

3. Provide information on the condition of the fetus or newborn.

Rationale: Keeping the patient informed will lessen her fear.

4. Provide information about the patient's own well-being, including vital signs, weight gain, and laboratory data.

Rationale: Such information may provide reassurance of personal well-being.

5. Encourage the presence of persons with whom the patient has important and positive relationships.

Rationale: Their presence may help the patient feel protected and secure.

Medical diagnosis

Medical diagnosis for placenta previa is based on ultrasound (to locate the implantation site of the placenta within the uterus).

Medical treatment

Treatment for placenta previa includes:

- hospitalization with bed rest
- no vaginal examination
- hematinic agents or blood transfusions to maintain a hematocrit level above 30%
- keeping two units of typed and crossmatched blood available at all times
- fetal surveillance testing using the nonstress test at least weekly (The contraction stress test is contraindicated because contractions may precipitate episodes of bleeding.)

• serial ultrasound for placental localization and fetal surveillance (The placenta is sometimes shifted away from the cervix as the uterus grows. Placenta previa is associated with increased incidence of fetal growth retardation and fetal anomalies.)
• $Rh_0(D)$ immune globulin if the woman is Rh-negative and has not been given the injection at 28 weeks' gestation
• Kleihauer-Betke test to detect excessive fetal-maternal hemorrhage
• cesarean section delivery, usually when fetal maturity is achieved or when the amount of bleeding is excessive or life-threatening.

☐ Postpartum hemorrhage (PPH)

Postpartum hemorrhage is defined as a blood loss exceeding 500 ml after delivery. Probably about 600 ml of blood is lost after most vaginal deliveries involving an episiotomy; because of the increase in blood volume during pregnancy, most women can tolerate this blood loss without complications. However, when blood loss approaches 1,000 ml, patients usually become symptomatic and treatment is necessary.

Early postpartum hemorrhage occurs during the first 24 hours after delivery and is usually caused by uterine atony, lacerations, or inversion of the uterus. Late postpartum hemorrhage refers to hemorrhage occurring after the first 24 hours and is usually caused by retained placental fragments. (See also "Disseminated intravascular coagulation" and "Hematoma" in this section.)

Predisposing factors include the following:
• overdistended uterus (twins, polyhydramnios, macrosomia)
• long labor
• oxytocin induction or augmentation
• urine retention
• precipitate labor
• placenta accreta
• operative delivery
• traction on the cord (uterine inversion)
• history of postpartum hemorrhage
• grand multiparity
• abruptio placentae
• general anesthesia
• clotting defects
• chorioamnionitis
• administration of magnesium sulfate.

Frequently encountered data for postpartum hemorrhage include the following:

Subjective data
• restlessness
• apprehension
• light-headedness

• nausea
• vision changes

Objective data
• massive vaginal bleeding
• boggy fundus (uterine atony)
• contracted uterus (laceration)
• increased pulse rate and decreased blood pressure (which may not change significantly until large amounts of blood have been lost)
• pallor and cool, moist skin
• chills
• no fundus or a dimple at the center of the fundus (uterine inversion).

   Below is a list of nursing diagnoses and interventions frequently associated with postpartum hemorrhage. (See also "Abruptio placentae," "Disseminated intravascular coagulation," "Hematoma," and "Placenta previa" in this section.)

Nursing diagnosis
Fluid Volume Deficit related to excessive blood loss
Desired outcome: Adequate tissue perfusion is maintained.

Nursing interventions and rationales
1. Administer I.V. fluids and blood replacement as ordered.
Rationale: This restores circulating blood volume.
2. Administer oxygen by face mask, as ordered.
Rationale: Giving oxygen increases oxygen saturation in blood.
3. Monitor the patient's vital signs closely.
Rationale: Such monitoring makes it possible to evaluate the cardiovascular effectiveness of blood circulation.
4. Monitor the patient's output hourly. An indwelling (Foley) catheter should be inserted.
Rationale: Urine output of 30 ml/hour indicates adequate renal perfusion.

Nursing diagnosis
Fluid Volume Excess related to rapid administration of oxytocin (which has antidiuretic properties)
Desired outcome: Normal blood volume is maintained.

Nursing interventions and rationales
1. Monitor the patient's central venous pressure (CVP) if a central venous line has been inserted.
Rationale: Increasing CVP indicates circulatory overload.
2. Auscultate the patient's lungs for crackles.
Rationale: Crackles may indicate impending pulmonary edema.
3. Monitor the patient's respiratory rate and effort.
Rationale: Increasing respiratory rate and dyspnea may signal impending pulmonary edema.

Nursing diagnosis
High Risk for Infection related to decreased resistance secondary to excessive blood loss
Desired outcome: No postpartum infection occurs.

Nursing interventions and rationales
1. Monitor the patient's temperature and pulse rate frequently.
Rationale: Increased temperature or pulse rate may indicate infection.
2. Monitor the patient's white blood cell count when ordered.
Rationale: An elevated white blood cell count may indicate infection, although it is somewhat elevated normally in the postpartum period.

Nursing diagnosis
Fear related to concern about excessive blood loss
Desired outcome: Patient and family are able to verbalize their concerns.

Nursing interventions and rationales
1. Keep the patient and her family informed regarding the patient's status and plan of care.
Rationale: Knowledge of the rationale and plan of care can be reassuring.
2. Allow a family member to remain with the patient if possible.
Rationale: The presence of a family member may decrease fear and anxiety.
3. Allow the patient and her family time to verbalize their feelings.
Rationale: Verbalization is therapeutic and helps the nurse to gain insight into their perceptions of the situation.

Medical diagnosis
Medical diagnosis for postpartum hemorrhage is based on:
• documentation of clinical signs and symptoms
• excessive bleeding with a boggy uterus, which may indicate atony
• excessive bleeding with a contracted uterus, which may indicate lacerations
• hemorrhage occurring 1 week to 10 days after delivery, which may be a sign of retained placental tissue
• a beefy-red mass presenting at the vaginal introitus, which may be a sign of uterine inversion.

Medical treatment
Treatment for postpartum hemorrhage includes:
• monitoring vital signs frequently
• administering oxygen
• inserting I.V. lines (an 18G needle should be used) capable of

administering blood and fluids rapidly, central venous pressure lines, or Swan-Ganz catheter in severe cases to accurately monitor cardiovascular status
• restoring circulating fluid volume with I.V. fluids and blood products (usually whole blood)
• prophylactic antibiotics (may be given because postpartum hemorrhage is associated with an increased incidence of infection

Uterine atony
• uterine massage to stimulate contractions
• bimanual uterine compression
• addition of 20 to 40 units of oxytocin in 1,000 ml of I.V. fluid
• administration of methergine or ergotrate if patient is not hypertensive
• prostaglandin F_{2a} (carboprost tromethamine), injected directly into the myometrium when previous measures have failed to control bleeding
• insertion of a CVP line or Swan-Ganz catheter in severe cases to monitor cardiovascular status more accurately
• laparotomy with hypogastric artery ligation or hysterectomy

Lacerations
• visualization of the site and suture

Retained placental fragments (usually a late cause of PPH)
• dilatation and curettage

Uterine inversion
• reinverting the uterus (anesthesia and tocolytic medications may be necessary to achieve relaxation)
• administration of oxytocic drugs to keep the uterus contracted.

☐ Post-term pregnancy

Pregnancies that extend past 294 days or 42 weeks are considered post-term or prolonged gestations. The perinatal mortality begins to increase after 42 weeks, doubles at 43 weeks, and is four to six times higher at 44 weeks than at term. The majority of pregnancies that extend beyond 42 weeks are actually a result of miscalculation of the expected date of confinement. However, because of the inaccuracy of ultrasound late in pregnancy, all pregnancies extending beyond 42 weeks must be monitored closely.

Predisposing factors include the following:
• anencephalic fetus
• fetal adrenal gland hypoplasia
• placental sulfatase deficiency
• extrauterine pregnancy (abdominal)
• previous post-term pregnancy
• male fetus.

Frequently encountered data for post-term pregnancy include the following:

Subjective data
• decreased fetal movement

Objective data
Prenatal

• oligohydramnios on ultrasound (The volume of amniotic fluid averages 300 ml at 42 weeks and decreases thereafter.)
• weight loss
• reduced rate of uterine growth
• fetal distress in labor (placental insufficiency caused by aging placenta; umbilical cord compression caused by decreased amniotic fluid)
• meconium-stained amniotic fluid

Neonatal

• profuse scalp hair
• long, thin body
• lack of subcutaneous fat
• parchment-like, peeling skin
• long fingernails
• lack of vernix
• meconium-stained skin, nails, and cord
• in some cases, continued growth and macrosomia
• wide-eyed appearance
• hypoglycemia
• temperature instability
• polycythemia.

Below is a nursing diagnosis with corresponding interventions and rationales frequently associated with post-term pregnancy. (See also "Birth trauma," "Hypoglycemia," and "Meconium aspiration syndrome" in this section.)

Nursing diagnosis
Fear related to prolonged pregnancy
Desired outcome: Patient will verbalize having less fear.

Nursing interventions and rationales
1. Explain to the patient the rationale for nonintervention and the purpose of fetal surveillance testing.
Rationale: Understanding the reason for allowing gestation to continue and the rationale behind testing decreases fear.
2. Allow the patient to verbalize her feeling regarding a prolonged pregnancy.
Rationale: Ventilation of feelings is therapeutic and serves as a basis for teaching.
3. Teach the patient to monitor fetal activity.
Rationale: Monitoring fetal activity allows the patient to become involved in her care and provides her with a means to measure fetal well-being between fetal surveillance tests.

Medical diagnosis
Medical diagnosis for post-term pregnancy is based on:
• accurate establishment of expected date of confinement using clinical parameters and early ultrasound examinations
• ultrasound for estimating amniotic fluid volume and ruling out fetal anomalies.

Medical treatment
Treatment for post-term pregnancy includes:
Prenatal
• induction of labor at 42 weeks if cervical status is compatible with induction and if the vertex is presenting and entering or in the maternal pelvis
• if cervical status is incompatible with induction, fetal surveillance testing beginning at 40 to 42 weeks using biweekly nonstress tests or contraction stress tests and ultrasound estimates of amniotic fluid volume (A biophysical profile has also been useful in identifying pregnancies at risk.)
• application of dinoprostone cervical gel to ripen the cervix prior to induction
• fetal monitoring during labor
• scalp pH for fetal distress
• proper suctioning for meconium-stained fluid at delivery
Newborn
• monitoring for hypoglycemia
• monitoring for meconium aspiration syndrome.

☐ Pregnancy-induced hypertension (PIH)
Also known as preeclampsia, PIH is a syndrome involving hypertension, edema, and proteinuria that develops after the 20th week of gestation. Severe PIH can progress to seizures (eclampsia).

Normal pregnant women are resistant to the pressor effects of angiotensin II, develop decreased peripheral resistance, and have increased blood volume. Women with PIH show an increased responsiveness to angiotensin II, increased peripheral resistance, and a constricted vascular space.

Although the cause of PIH is unknown, generalized vasospasms are thought to be responsible for much of the pathology of the disease. Abruptio placentae, disseminated intravascular coagulation, thrombocytopenia, placental insufficiency, and intrauterine fetal death are associated complications.

Predisposing factors include the following:
• primigravida
• low socioeconomic status
• poor nutrition
• age (teenagers and women over age 35)
• previous PIH

- chronic hypertension
- diabetes
- twins
- hydatidiform mole
- family history (mother or sister with PIH)
- hydrops fetalis
- polyhydramnios
- chronic renal disease.

Frequently encountered data for PIH include the following:

Subjective data
- headache
- vision changes
- vertigo
- scotomata (spots before the eyes)
- nausea
- heartburn, right upper quadrant pain (swelling of the liver capsule)

Objective data
- elevated blood pressure (blood pressure greater than 140/90 mm Hg or a rise of 30 mm Hg systolic or 15 mm Hg diastolic from the patient's usual blood pressure)
- edema involving the face and hands
- proteinuria
- vomiting
- rapid weight gain
- hyperactive reflexes with or without clonus
- increased hematocrit level
- decreased renal output
- hematuria.

Below is a list of nursing diagnoses and interventions frequently associated with PIH. (See also "Abruptio placentae," "Disseminated intravascular coagulation," and "Intrauterine growth retardation" in this section.)

Nursing diagnosis
Altered Systemic Tissue Perfusion related to generalized vasospasms
Desired outcome: Adequate oxygenation of tissues is maintained.

Nursing interventions and rationales
1. Encourage the patient to maintain bed rest in the lateral position.
Rationale: Bed rest in this position increases uteroplacental blood flow.
2. Perform fetal surveillance testing (nonstress test or contraction stress test), as ordered.
Rationale: These tests make it possible to evaluate placental efficiency in providing the fetus with oxygen and nutrients.
3. Monitor the patient's vital signs closely.

Rationale: Progression of hypertension further decreases tissue perfusion.

4. Monitor the patient's fluid intake and output.

Rationale: Urine output of 30 ml/hour indicates adequate renal perfusion.

5. Administer medications, as ordered, to lower the patient's blood pressure.

Rationale: Severe hypertension can cause a cerebrovascular accident. Blood pressure should not be lowered drastically because placental perfusion can be compromised.

6. Monitor the patient's neurologic status.

Rationale: Changes in neurologic status can indicate cerebral hypoxia or impending seizure activity.

7. Monitor I.V. fluids closely. Avoid rapid infusion of I.V. fluids.

Rationale: Vascular space is vasoconstricted; rapid infusion of fluids can cause pulmonary edema.

Nursing diagnosis
High Risk for Injury: Hypoxia related to seizures
Desired outcome: Patient will experience no seizures or the injury they can cause.

Nursing interventions and rationales
1. Assess for signs of worsening PIH or impending seizure (blood pressure of 160/110 mm Hg or above, epigastric pain, decreased urine output, visual changes, headache, excessive proteinuria).

Rationale: Prompt treatment can prevent seizure activity.

2. Provide a calm, nonstimulating environment.

Rationale: This decreases central nervous system stimulation.

3. Institute seizure precautions (raising side rails and keeping a tongue depressor, oxygen, and suction available).

Rationale: These precautions can help you provide rapid treatment if seizure occurs.

4. Administer medications as ordered.

Rationale: Medication may help to prevent seizure activity.

5. Monitor the patient for deep tendon reflexes and for the presence of clonus.

Rationale: Hyperreflexia indicates increased central nervous system irritability.

Medical diagnosis
Medical diagnosis for PIH is based on documentation of clinical signs and symptoms; serum uric acid levels are elevated in PIH but not in chronic hypertension.

Medical treatment
Treatment for PIH includes:

Mild preeclampsia (minimal blood pressure elevation)
• bed rest in the lateral position

• adequate fluid intake
• increased protein in the diet
• regular sodium in the diet with no added salt
• checking for deep tendon reflexes and clonus (See "Deep tendon reflexes" in Section 3.)
• monitoring the patient's progress closely; seeing the patient twice a week if she is not hospitalized
• twice-weekly nonstress tests or contraction stress tests
• ultrasound for monitoring fetal growth
• monitoring coagulation studies
• monitoring weight gain

Severe preeclampsia (delivery is indicated)
• administration of magnesium sulfate
• administration of hydralazine 5 to 10 mg I.V. slowly for diastolic pressures of 110 mm Hg or greater (aimed at preventing cerebrovascular accident)
• inserting a central venous pressure line or Swan-Ganz catheter for hemodynamic monitoring
• induction of labor if cervix is favorable (vaginal delivery is preferable to cesarean section)
• continued administration of magnesium sulfate for 24 to 48 hours postpartum
Note: Use of epidural anesthesia is controversial (see "Epidural block" in Section 3).

Eclampsia
• protecting the patient from injury
• stopping seizures with medications (magnesium sulfate, valium, amobarbital sodium)
• delivery after stabilization.

☐ Premature rupture of the membranes (PROM)

Premature rupture of the membranes occurs before the onset of labor. The primary risk to the mother is infection. Potential fetal and neonatal complications include anoxia, breech or transverse lie, cord prolapse, preterm delivery, respiratory distress syndrome, sepsis, and traumatic delivery.

About 80% of patients at term go into labor within 24 hours of rupture, whereas only 50% of those with preterm gestations go into labor spontaneously within the same period. Tocolytics are usually contraindicated in PROM. (See also "Chorioamnionitis," "Endometritis," and "Preterm labor" in this section.)

Predisposing factors include the following:
• polyhydramnios
• chorioamnionitis
• vaginal infection
• low socioeconomic status
• incompetent cervix

- placenta previa
- genetic anomalies
- malpresentation
- multiple gestation
- trauma.

Frequently encountered data for premature rupture of the membranes include the following:

Subjective data
- feeling of wetness

Objective data
- vaginal pooling of fluid seen on pelvic examination
- decreased amniotic fluid on ultrasound
- positive nitrazine test (see "Nitrazine test" in Section 3)
- positive fern test (see "Fern test" in Section 3).

For a list of nursing diagnoses and interventions frequently associated with premature rupture of the membranes, see "Chorioamnionitis," "Endometritis," "Preterm labor," and "Sepsis" in this section.

Medical diagnosis

Medical diagnosis for premature rupture of the membranes is based on:
- visual detection of amniotic fluid escaping from the cervical os or of vaginal pooling of amniotic fluid
- positive nitrazine and fern test
- ultrasound for amniotic fluid level.

Medical treatment

Treatment for premature rupture of the membranes includes:

Conservative therapy (with no evidence of infection)
- monitoring temperature and pulse rate every 2 to 4 hours
- listening to fetal heart tones every 4 to 8 hours
- obtaining a complete blood count with differential
- using a nonstress test or biophysical profile to maintain fetal status
- monitoring for uterine tenderness
- amniocentesis for bacterial and white blood cell counts (has been advocated as a method of determining which patients should be managed more aggressively)

Aggressive therapy (with evidence of infection or fetal jeopardy)
- induction of labor (see "Induction of labor" in Section 3)
- cesarean section for obstetric indications.

☐ Preterm birth

A preterm birth refers to one that occurs before 37 completed weeks of gestation. Most premature newborns weigh less than 5 lb, 8 oz (2,500 g) and are poorly equipped to handle the stresses of extrauterine life.

For example, a premature infant lacks adequate lung surfactant, which can result in respiratory distress syndrome. His immature digestive tract will have difficulty absorbing fats and other nutrients; asphyxial episodes can lead to necrotizing enterocolitis. His immune system will be incapable of fighting infection, and his immature central nervous system and the lack of subcutaneous fat will lead to temperature instability. Also, capillary fragility in the brain will predispose him to intraventricular hemorrhage. (See also "Hyperbilirubinemia," "Hypoglycemia," "Respiratory distress syndrome," and "Sepsis" in this section).

Predisposing factors include the following:
• history of premature delivery
• multiple gestation
• lack of prenatal care
• incompetent cervix
• chorioamnionitis
• premature rupture of the membranes
• failed tocolysis
• contraindication to tocolytic therapy
• placenta previa
• pregnancy-induced hypertension
• medical or obstetric indication for delivery
• iatrogenic causes (induced inadvertently by health care provider or treatment).

Frequently encountered data include the following:

Subjective data
Not applicable

Objective data
• lack of subcutaneous fat
• temperature instability
• poor muscle tone
• poor sucking reflex
• respiratory distress
• hypoglycemia, hyperbilirubinemia
• birth weight less than 5 lb, 8 oz (2,500 g). (Infants of diabetic patients may weigh more than 5 lb, 8 oz and still be premature.)

Below is a list of nursing diagnoses and interventions frequently associated with premature births. (See also "Hyperbilirubinemia," "Hypoglycemia," and "Sepsis" in this section).

Nursing diagnosis
Ineffective Thermoregulation related to lack of subcutaneous fat and to central nervous system immaturity
Desired outcome: The newborn's temperature normalizes.

Nursing interventions and rationales
1. Avoid exposing the newborn to heat loss from evaporation, convection, conduction, and radiation.

Rationale: These are mechanisms whereby the newborn can develop hypothermia.
2. Monitor the newborn's skin temperature.
Rationale: Monitoring provides necessary continuous information regarding temperature status.
3. Monitor the heating unit for correct temperature and proper functioning.
Rationale: An external heating unit is necessary to maintain a neutral thermal environment.

Nursing diagnosis
Anticipatory Grieving related to threatened loss of infant and failure to produce a perfect child
Desired outcome: Parent-infant attachment occurs and parents understand the rationale for the grieving process.

Nursing interventions and rationales
1. Provide the parents with adequate, realistic information about the infant's condition and prognosis.
Rationale: Providing correct information may help the grieving process and may prevent a false sense of security.
2. Encourage the parents to have frequent contact with the infant.
Rationale: Frequent contact facilitates attachment. Premature newborns suffer a higher incidence of child abuse, probably because of a failure of attachment.
3. Allow the parents time to verbalize their feelings and fears about the premature birth.
Rationale: Verbalization is therapeutic and helps the nurse identify the need for further counseling.
4. Refer the parents to appropriate support groups.
Rationale: Comfort and reassurance can be obtained from parents who have experienced a similar crisis.

Medical diagnosis
Medical diagnosis for preterm birth is based on:
• measuring birth weight
• clinical appearance and symptoms
• gestational age assessment.

Medical treatment
Treatment for preterm birth is as follows:
• maintaining a neutral thermal environment
• monitoring for hypoglycemia
• monitoring for respiratory distress
• administering I.V. fluids to maintain fluid and electrolyte balance
• gavage feeding if sucking is poor or requires excessive physical effort
• Total parenteral nutrition, if necessary

• monitoring serum bilirubin levels.
Note: For treatments of specific disorders listed under predisposing factors above, see the corresponding entries in this section.

☐ Preterm labor

Preterm labor is defined as labor that begins after the 20th week and before the 37th completed week of gestation. Preterm birth is the leading cause of early neonatal death; many survivors suffer significant developmental handicaps. Drugs available for treating preterm labor have been relatively unsuccessful in altering the prematurity rate. Prenatal screening tools, such as weekly cervical examinations for those at risk and home monitoring for uterine activity, are aimed at diagnosis earlier in the pregnancy, when tocolytic drugs can be used more successfully.

Predisposing factors include the following:
• incompetent cervix
• multiple gestation
• premature rupture of the membranes
• chorioamnionitis
• placenta previa
• polyhydramnios
• pyelonephritis
• maternal age less than 18 years
• poor nutrition
• smoking
• previous preterm labor
• previous second trimester abortion
• uterine anomalies
• abdominal surgery during pregnancy.

Frequently encountered data for preterm labor include the following:

Subjective data
• increased or bloody discharge
• backache
• pressure, cramping
• contractions

Objective data
• diarrhea
• cervical change (effacement, dilation of anterior cervix, ballooning of the lower segment into the vagina)
• palpable uterine contractions or contractions evident on external monitor.

Below is a list of nursing diagnoses and interventions frequently associated with preterm labor. (See also "Multiple gestation," "Placenta previa," "Premature rupture of the membranes," and "Pyelonephritis" in this section.)

Nursing diagnosis

High Risk for Maternal Injury related to side effects of tocolytic therapy
Desired outcome: No complications from tocolytic drugs occur.

Nursing interventions and rationales

1. Monitor vital signs frequently.
Rationale: Hypotension can occur. Pulse rates greater than 140 beats/minute are associated with the development of pulmonary edema. Pulse rates less than 100 beats/minute may indicate an ineffective dose. Increased respiratory rate may indicate impending pulmonary edema.
2. Monitor fetal heart tones.
Rationale: Tachycardia is common. Fetal distress is a contraindication to tocolysis.
3. Auscultate lungs every 4 hours.
Rationale: Crackles may indicate impending pulmonary edema.
4. Monitor I.V. fluids carefully.
Rationale: Fluid overload can precipitate pulmonary edema.

5. Monitor for chest pain and cardiac arrhythmias.
Rationale: Myocardial ischemia has been reported.

Nursing diagnosis

Ineffective Individual Coping related to prolonged bed rest and side effects of medications
Desired outcome: Patient adjusts satisfactorily to restrictions imposed by the diagnosis.

Nursing interventions and rationales

1. Encourage the patient's verbalization of feelings about the diagnosis and about restrictions imposed on physical activity.
Rationale: Verbalization can be therapeutic and serves as a basis for teaching and counseling.
2. Explain to the patient the rationale for the plan of care, and discuss the problems related to prematurity.
Rationale: The patient's understanding of the reason behind the treatment and the complications that can result from premature labor should increase patient compliance.
3. Encourage the patient to use support systems, such as family and friends, in meeting her needs and the needs of her family.
Rationale: The patient may be unable to perform total care for the family because of medical restrictions.
4. Obtain a social service consultation, if necessary.
Rationale: Financial and personal obligations may be a source of considerable stress to the patient.

Nursing diagnosis

Fear related to the possibility of preterm delivery
Desired outcome: Patient expresses confidence in the plan of care.

Nursing interventions and rationales

1. Keep the patient and family informed regarding test results, fetal status, and any need for alterations in the care plan.
Rationale: Patients are less fearful if they know what to expect and are kept abreast of the progress in their treatment.
2. Teach the patient to monitor for contractions and fetal activity. (Some centers are now using home monitoring by telephone to identify uterine activity.)
Rationale: Such monitoring involves the patient in her care and provides her with some element of control.
3. Provide appropriate reassurance.
Rationale: The patient's or her family's perceptions of the situation may be unrealistically negative.

Medical diagnosis

Medical diagnosis for preterm labor is based on:
• contractions occurring at least once every 10 minutes and lasting 30 seconds or longer
• documented cervical change or cervical effacement of 80% or dilatation of 2 cm.

Medical treatment

Treatment for preterm labor includes:
• hydration with I.V. therapy
• sedation
• bed rest in the left lateral position
• treatment of urinary tract infection or pyelonephritis if present (see "Pyelonephritis" in this section)
• tocolytic therapy until the 36th to 37th week of gestation
• administration of betamethasone to stimulate fetal lung maturity when preterm delivery appears inevitable

☐ Prolapsed cord

Prolapse of the umbilical cord in front of the presenting part is considered an emergency in obstetrics. Such prolapse compresses the cord between the presenting part and the bony pelvis and shuts off fetal circulation.

In many cases, prolapse follows rupture of the membranes. The nurse must be diligent in observing the patient for signs and symptoms of cord prolapse after spontaneous or induced membrane rupture. (See "Amniotomy" in Section 3 and *Prolapse of the umbilical cord*, page 144.)

Predisposing factors include the following:
• malpresentations
• cephalopelvic disproportion
• abnormal fetal positioning
• prematurity
• lack of engagement of the presenting part.

PROLAPSE OF THE UMBILICAL CORD

If the umbilical cord falls level with or below the fetus' presenting part, consider it prolapsed. If the fetus' presenting part presses the cord against the mother's pelvis, the blood and oxygen supply is cut off. Fetal neurologic damage or death may result.

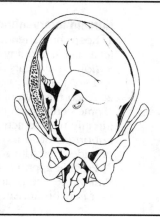

Frequently encountered data for a prolapsed cord include the following:

Subjective data
• a feeling that something is coming through the vagina

Objective data
• variable decelerations or bradycardia after rupture of the membranes
• palpation of the cord on vaginal examination or prolapse of the cord out of the vagina.

Below is a list of nursing diagnoses and interventions frequently associated with prolapse of the umbilical cord. (See also "Cesarean section" in this section.)

Nursing diagnosis

Impaired Gas Exchange related to altered oxygen supply to the fetus caused by cord compression
Desired outcome: Adequate tissue oxygenation is maintained.

Nursing interventions and rationales

1. Lift the presenting part off the cord (by applying finger pressure against the presenting part or placing the patient in a modified Sims' position) until cesarean section can be performed.
Rationale: This measure relieves cord compression and restores blood flow through the cord.
2. Administer oxygen to the patient, as ordered.
Rationale: Increased maternal oxygen saturation provides more oxygen to the fetus.

Nursing diagnosis

Fear related to the emergency and to the possible death of the fetus
Desired outcome: Patient verbalizes that her fear is reduced.

Nursing interventions and rationales
1. Remain calm (labor room personnel should remain calm but efficient in handling the emergency).
Rationale: Fear is reduced when the patient feels confident about the health care team.
2. Allow family members to remain at the bedside if possible.
Rationale: The presence of a support person may lessen anxiety.
3. Explain what is happening and why as the patient is prepared for operative delivery.
Rationale: Conversing with the patient while she is being prepared for delivery will lessen her anxiety.

Medical diagnosis
Medical diagnosis is based on clinical signs and symptoms.

Medical treatment
Treatment for prolapsed cord includes:
• elevating the presenting part off the umbilical cord
• immediate delivery by cesarean section.

☐ Pyelonephritis
Associated with an increased incidence of anemia, low-birth-weight newborns, pregnancy-induced hypertension, premature labor and delivery, and premature rupture of the membranes, pyelonephritis results directly from bacterial infection that extends upward from the bladder through the blood vessels and lymphatics.

Acute pyelonephritis most frequently follows untreated or inadequately treated urinary tract infection or asymptomatic bacteriuria. About 30% of patients with these conditions subsequently develop symptomatic pyelonephritis, usually during the third trimester.

Predisposing factors include the following:
• urinary tract infections
• asymptomatic bacteriuria
• sickle cell trait
• anatomic defects of the urinary tract
• obstructive and neurologic diseases of the urinary tract
• renal calculi.

Frequently encountered data for pyelonephritis include the following:

Subjective data
• flank pain
• burning or painful urination
• increased frequency of urination
• chills
• malaise
• nausea

Objective data
- increased temperature, pulse rate, and fetal heart tones
- elevated white blood cell count
- more than 100,000 colonies of bacteria/milliliter of urine
- uterine contractions
- vomiting.

Below is a nursing diagnosis with appropriate interventions and rationales frequently associated with pyelonephritis. (See also "Preterm labor" and "Urinary tract infection" in this section.)

Nursing diagnosis
High Risk for Injury related to complications of pyelonephritis (such as preterm labor and renal damage)
Desired outcome: No complications occur.

Nursing interventions and rationales
1. Monitor for contractions, and instruct the patient on how to monitor for uterine activity and for other signs of preterm labor.
Rationale: Early identification of preterm labor increases the success of treatment.
2. Instruct the patient regarding the importance of compliance in taking antibiotics and in making and keeping follow-up appointments.
Rationale: Chronic pyelonephritis can cause renal damage. Completing the prescribed antibiotic course will decrease the incidence of relapse.

Medical diagnosis
Medical diagnosis is based on:
- clinical signs and symptoms
- pyuria and bacteriuria on urinalysis
- urine culture, more than 100,000 colonies of bacteria/milliliter of urine.

Medical treatment
Treatment for pyelonephritis includes:
- administration of I.V. antibiotics
- hydration
- administration of antipyretics (acetaminophen)
- monitoring of renal function
- monitoring of fluid intake and output
- urine cultures every 2 to 4 weeks after resolution of the infection
- possible chronic suppression for the duration of the pregnancy (administering 100 mg of nitrofurantoin every night)
- intravenous pyelogram 6 weeks postpartum to identify upper urinary tract disease.

☐ Respiratory distress syndrome (RDS)

Normal surfactant production and, therefore, normal pulmonary function occur at about 35 weeks of gestation. Deficiencies in surfactant, a substance that prevents the alveoli from collapsing on expiration, can lead to respiratory distress syndrome (RDS Type I) in the newborn. (RDS Type II, also known as transient tachypnea of the newborn, is discussed in "Transient tachypnea of the newborn" in this section.)

With RDS, every breath the newborn takes is like the initial breath at delivery, requiring considerable energy and effort to inflate the alveoli. As the newborn's reserves dissipate, atelectasis and pulmonary hypoperfusion develop. Hypoxia, hypercapnea, and metabolic and respiratory acidosis ensue. Persistent fetal circulation develops as a result of hypoperfusion of the lungs.

Predisposing factors include the following:
- prematurity
- maternal diabetes
- intrauterine asphyxia
- cesarean delivery
- lecithin-sphingomyelin ratio less than 2:1
- absence of phosphatidylglycerol in amniotic fluid.

Frequently encountered data for respiratory distress syndrome include the following:

Subjective data
Not applicable

Objective data
- tachypnea
- flaring nares
- expiratory grunting
- retractions
- pallor, cyanosis
- decreased breath sounds
- crepitant crackles
- apneic episodes
- edema
- hypothermia
- poor muscle tone.

Below is a list of nursing diagnoses and interventions frequently associated with RDS.

Nursing diagnosis
Impaired Gas Exchange related to atelectasis, persistent fetal circulation, and poor respiratory effort
Desired outcome: Blood gas measurements and blood pH remain within normal limits.

Nursing interventions and rationales
1. Monitor blood gas measurements and arterial pH levels as ordered.

Rationale: Monitoring helps to determine the effectiveness of or the need for alteration in therapy.

2. Administer oxygen as ordered.

Rationale: Supplemental oxygen increases the supply available for exchange.

3. Administer continuous positive airway pressure (CPAP) or ventilatory assistance and positive end-expiratory pressure (PEEP), as ordered.

Rationale: These measures maintain expansion of the alveoli on expiration, which improves ventilation.

4. Observe the newborn's color, respiratory rate, and degree of effort involved in breathing (if he is not on a ventilator); auscultate his lungs frequently.

Rationale: Changes in respiratory status may indicate a worsening of the newborn's condition and may necessitate a change in therapy.

Nursing diagnosis
Ineffective Airway Clearance related to increased secretions and inability to cough
Desired outcome: No mucus accumulation occurs to impede air flow in the lungs.

Nursing interventions and rationales
1. Suction the newborn, as needed.

Rationale: Suctioning removes secretions.

2. Observe the newborn's tolerance of suctioning. (Check his color and heart rate, as well as the amount, character, and color of secretions.)

Rationale: Suctioning can be traumatic to the newborn, causing increased respiratory difficulty and induced bradycardia from vagal stimulation.

3. Alter the newborn's position frequently. Use postural chest drainage as ordered.

Rationale: These measures prevent stasis of secretions and aid in their removal.

4. Maintain adequate hydration.

Rationale: Adequate hydration prevents thick secretions, which are harder to remove.

Nursing diagnosis
High Risk for Fluid Volume Deficit or Excess related to disease process, fluid loss, and I.V. administration
Desired outcome: Fluid and electrolyte balance is maintained.

Nursing interventions and rationales
1. Weigh the newborn daily.

Rationale: Weighing helps to evaluate body fluid balance.

2. Monitor laboratory values.

Rationale: Laboratory values serve as a guide for replacement therapy.

3. Observe for signs and symptoms of fluid and electrolyte imbalance.

Rationale: The newborn's condition can change rapidly; prompt recognition and treatment minimizes complications.

4. Administer and monitor I.V. fluids carefully.

Rationale: Fluid imbalances can develop rapidly from an increase or decrease in I.V. fluids.

Nursing diagnosis

Altered Nutrition: Less Than Body Requirements related to large caloric expenditure and low nutritional intake
Desired outcome: Infant's weight stabilizes and he begins to gain.

Nursing interventions and rationales

1. Minimize the newborn's caloric expenditure by means of neutral thermal environment, gavage feeding, and respiratory support.

Rationale: Avoiding unnecessary caloric expenditure conserves calories for growth.

2. Monitor the newborn's weight daily.

Rationale: Weight monitoring helps to evaluate the therapy used.

3. Provide nutrition as ordered. (Higher caloric formulas in small, frequent amounts are often used for preterm infants.)

Rationale: Added nutrition supplies calories for growth.

4. Elevate the head of the bed after feeding.

Rationale: The newborn's cardiac sphincter is poorly developed; regurgitation occurs frequently.

Nursing diagnosis

High Risk for Injury related to treatment for RDS
Desired outcome: Infant develops no pulmonary complications from treatment for RDS.

Nursing interventions and rationales

1. Observe the newborn for signs and symptoms of pneumothorax.

Rationale: CPAP can cause pneumothorax because of increased pressures within the lungs.

2. Monitor the newborn's oxygen concentrations frequently.

Rationale: High oxygen concentrations over prolonged intervals can cause retinopathy of prematurity (formerly known as retrolental fibroplasia).

3. Monitor the newborn's bowel sounds and stools for abnormal findings.

Rationale: Necrotizing enterocolitis is seen more frequently in infants with RDS.

4. Monitor the newborn's neurologic status.

Rationale: Intraventricular hemorrhage is seen more frequently in infants with RDS.

5. Monitor for signs of persistent fetal circulation.

Rationale: RDS often precipitates persistent fetal circulation.

6. Observe for the development of bronchopulmonary dysplasia.

Rationale: This chronic lung disorder is a possible result of prolonged ventilatory support.

Other nursing diagnoses

Other nursing diagnoses associated with respiratory distress syndrome include the following:

• Altered Family Processes related to stress of having one's child in the neonatal intensive care unit

• High Risk for Altered Parenting related to prolonged hospitalization of the newborn

• Anticipatory Grieving related to the possibility of death of the newborn

• Knowledge Deficit: Parental related to poor understanding of the disease process

Medical diagnosis

Medical diagnosis for RDS is based on:

• blood gas measurements (decreased PO_2, increased PCO_2, decreased pH)

• chest X-ray

• clinical signs and symptoms.

Medical treatment

Treatment for RDS includes:

Assisted ventilation

• oxygen administration

• CPAP to provide positive pressure at end-expiration, which maintains distention of alveoli on expiration

• surfactant replacement therapy via the endotracheal tube

• mechanical ventilation

• extracorporeal membrane oxygenation (ECMO)

Other procedures

• I.V. therapy

• correcting metabolic acidosis

• maintaining a neutral thermal environment

• maintaining blood pressure

• packed red blood cells to maintain a normal hematocrit level.

☐ Sepsis (neonatal)

This condition usually refers to a generalized infection characterized by proliferation of bacteria in the bloodstream. The newborn is vulnerable to infection because of an immature immune system and the loss of the protective environment of the uterus. The fetus can become infected in utero, during passage through the birth canal at delivery, or from exposure after birth.

Predisposing factors include the following:
• chorioamnionitis
• prolonged rupture of the membranes
• preterm birth
• presence of maternal infection.

Frequently encountered data for neonatal sepsis include the following:

Subjective data
Not applicable

Objective data
• bulging fontanelle
• lethargy, hypotonia
• jitteriness, irritability
• temperature instability (usually hypothermia)
• tremors, seizures
• poor feeding
• vomiting, diarrhea
• skin rash
• jaundice
• apnea, tachypnea
• cyanosis
• grunting
• thrombocytopenia, leukopenia, disseminated intravascular coagulation
• abdominal distention
• hypoglycemia.

Below is a list of nursing diagnoses and interventions frequently associated with sepsis. (See also "Hyperbilirubinemia," "Hypoglycemia," and "Respiratory distress syndrome" in this section.)

Nursing diagnosis
High Risk for Fluid Volume Deficit related to vomiting, diarrhea, or poor feeding
Desired outcome: Fluid balance is maintained.

Nursing interventions and rationales
1. Weigh the newborn daily.
Rationale: Weighing helps to evaluate fluid balance.
2. Monitor the newborn's fluid intake and output.
Rationale: Monitoring helps to evaluate fluid balance and serves as a guide for fluid replacement.
3. Monitor the newborn's serum electrolyte levels, as ordered.
Rationale: Loss of fluid often results in electrolyte imbalance.
4. Administer oral or I.V. fluids, as ordered.

Rationale: Additional fluids may restore and maintain blood volume.
5. Monitor the newborn's vital signs.
Rationale: Decreased blood pressure and increased pulse rate are signs of dehydration.

Nursing diagnosis
Altered Cardiopulmonary Tissue Perfusion related to hypotension
Desired outcome: Adequate cardiac output and tissue perfusion are maintained.

Nursing interventions and rationales
1. Monitor the newborn's vital signs frequently.
Rationale: Subtle changes can indicate a deterioration in the newborn.
2. Monitor the newborn's arterial blood gas levels.
Rationale: Monitoring of arterial blood gas levels helps to evaluate tissue perfusion to the lungs.
3. Administer medications, as ordered, to maintain the newborn's blood pressure.
Rationale: Vasopressors may be needed to maintain tissue perfusion.
4. Monitor the newborn's fluid intake and output.
Rationale: Such monitoring helps to evaluate fluid balance. Adequate urine output indicates sufficient renal perfusion.
5. Administer oxygen, as ordered.
Rationale: Administering oxygen helps to maximize arterial oxygenation.
6. Administer I.V. fluids and blood products, as ordered.
Rationale: These measures help to maintain circulating volume.

Nursing diagnosis
High Risk for Infection related to immature immune system
Desired outcome: Risk of infection is minimized; if infection occurs, infection is identified and treated promptly. Nosocomial infections do not occur.

Nursing interventions and rationales
1. Perform strict hand washing when handling infants; follow universal precautions.
Rationale: These actions prevent transmission of infection from health care personnel to infants and from infant to infant.
2. Monitor vital signs, color, tone, and feeding patterns.
Rationale: Temperature instability, respiratory distress, tachycardia, pallor, cyanosis, hypotonia, and a poor sucking reflex can be signs of sepsis.
3. Administer antibiotics on time as ordered for suspected or actual infections.
Rationale: Maintenance of therapeutic antibiotic blood levels is essential for treatment.

Other nursing diagnoses
• High Risk for Altered Parenting related to separation of parents and infant
• Interrupted Breast-feeding related to prolonged hospitalization of the newborn.

Medical diagnosis
Medical diagnosis for neonatal sepsis is based on:
• positive cultures (blood, skin, cerebrospinal fluid)
• increased sedimentation rate
• thrombocytopenia, leukopenia, disseminated intravascular coagulation
• clinical signs and symptoms.

Medical treatment
Treatment for neonatal sepsis includes:
• administration of antibiotics
• symptomatic treatment of shock, metabolic acidosis, and renal failure.

☐ Thrombophlebitis
An inflammatory process of the lining of a vein associated with formation of a thrombus, thrombophlebitis often precedes pulmonary embolism.
   Predisposing factors include the following:
• operative delivery
• history of thrombophlebitis
• obesity
• hemorrhage
• varicosities
• anemia
• heart disease
• prolonged labor
• pregnancy-induced hypertension
• endometritis
• diabetes
• maternal age over 35
• prolonged immobilization.
   Frequently encountered data for thrombophlebitis include the following:

Subjective data
• pain in the affected extremity
• chills

Objective data
• edema
• erythema
• positive Homans' sign

• elevated temperature and increased pulse.

Below is a list of nursing diagnoses and interventions frequently associated with thrombophlebitis.

Nursing diagnosis

Altered Peripheral Tissue Perfusion related to changes in the blood vessels secondary to the disease process
Desired outcome: No permanent tissue damage occurs.

Nursing interventions and rationales

1. Apply warmth and moisture to the extremity, as ordered.
Rationale: Warmth and moisture increase blood flow to the area and may reduce edema and inflammation.
2. Promote bed rest and limited activity of the extremity.
Rationale: Rest reduces tissue energy requirements and may prevent thrombi from dislodging in vessels.
3. Teach the patient to avoid smoking and environmental factors that promote vasoconstriction, such as exposure to the cold.
Rationale: Vasoconstriction diminishes blood flow to tissues.
4. Observe the patient for signs of respiratory distress or chest pain.
Rationale: Emboli may dislodge and travel to the lung.
5. Administer anticoagulants, as ordered.
Rationale: Anticoagulants decrease the formation of clots within the vascular system.

Nursing diagnosis

Pain related to tissue ischemia and inflammation
Desired outcome: Pain is reduced or eliminated.

Nursing interventions and rationales

1. Institute measures to increase circulation to the patient's extremity, including heat application, avoiding cold and smoking, and limiting activity.
Rationale: Improved tissue perfusion reduces pain.
2. Change the patient's position frequently, and offer back rubs and other comfort measures.
Rationale: Prolonged bed rest can cause discomfort from pressure and stiffness of joints.
3. Administer analgesics, as ordered.
Rationale: Central nervous system depressants minimize pain.

Nursing diagnosis

High Risk for Injury related to bleeding secondary to treatment for thrombophlebitis
Desired outcome: No complications occur during treatment.

Nursing interventions and rationales
1. Observe the patient for bleeding.
Rationale: Anticoagulant therapy predisposes the patient to bleeding.
2. Monitor the patient's prothrombin time or partial thromboplastin time (depending on use of warfarin or heparin therapy), as ordered.
Rationale: These laboratory tests help to evaluate the effectiveness of therapy and to prevent overdose.
3. Monitor the patient's platelet count, as ordered.
Rationale: Some patients develop thrombocytopenia with heparin use.

Nursing diagnosis
Diversional Activity Deficit related to prolonged bed rest
Desired outcome: Patient expresses interest in using time meaningfully.

Nursing interventions and rationales
1. Explain to the patient the rationale for treatment and the need for prolonged bed rest.
Rationale: Understanding the reason for the imposed restriction will increase patient compliance.
2. Encourage the patient's family to bring in familiar objects, such as photographs, and to provide diversional activities, such as needlepoint and reading materials, for the patient.
Rationale: Familiar objects and enjoyable activities may help the patient feel more comfortable and may divert her focus from her complication.
3. Provide a compatible roommate for the patient.
Rationale: Companionship helps prevent the depression that may be caused by hospitalization.

Other nursing diagnoses
Other nursing diagnoses associated with thrombophlebitis include:
• Altered Family Processes related to prolonged hospitalization
• Impaired Home Maintenance Management related to limited activity
• Knowledge Deficit related to disease, treatment, and potential complications.

Medical diagnosis
Medical diagnosis for thrombophlebitis is based on:
• Doppler ultrasound studies
• plethysmography

• venography (involves radiation exposure to fetus)
• ^{125}I-fibrinogen scanning (involves radiation exposure to fetus).

Medical treatment
Treatment for thrombophlebitis includes:
• bed rest
• elevation of, and application of heat to, the affected extremity
• use of support hose
• anticoagulation with heparin.

☐ Transient tachypnea of the newborn

Transient tachypnea of the newborn (TTN), also known as respiratory distress syndrome Type II, may occur in preterm or term newborns. The major clinical finding is delayed reabsorption of fetal lung fluid. In contrast to respiratory distress syndrome Type I, the prognosis for newborns with TTN is generally good.

Frequently encountered data for TTN include the following:

Subjective data
Not applicable

Objective data
• tachypnea
• excessive oropharyngeal secretions
• retractions
• flaring nares
• barrel chest
• expiratory grunt
• cyanosis in room air
• generalized overexpansion of the lungs on X-ray.

For a list of nursing diagnoses and interventions frequently associated with TTN, see "Respiratory distress syndrome" in this section.

Medical diagnosis
Medical diagnosis of TTN is based on:
• clinical signs and symptoms
• chest X-ray.

Medical treatment
Treatment for TTN includes:
• oxygen by hood
• close observation for signs of sepsis. (The clinical course of Group B streptococcal pneumonia is identical to that of TTN for the first 12 to 24 hours.)
Note: The condition usually resolves in 6 to 24 hours but may last as long as 4 days in asphyxiated infants.

☐ Urinary tract infection (UTI)

The most common medical complication of pregnancy, UTIs may be either asymptomatic (asymptomatic bacteriuria of pregnancy, or ASB) or symptomatic (cystitis). Of women with untreated ASB, 20% to 40% develop pyelonephritis.

Predisposing factors for UTI include the following:
* anatomic defects of the urinary tract
* sickle cell trait
* poor hygiene
* history of UTI or pyelonephritis
* anemia
* diabetes
* normal changes of the urinary tract found in pregnant women.
Frequently encountered data for UTI include the following:

Subjective data
* burning and pain on urination
* lower abdominal pain
* increased frequency of urination
* costovertebral angle tenderness

Objective data
* fever
* positive nitrates on dipstick
* proteinuria, hematuria, bacteriuria, white blood cells in urine.

Below is a list of nursing diagnoses and interventions frequently associated with UTI. (See also "Pyelonephritis" in this section.)

Nursing diagnosis
Pain related to infection
Desired outcome: Pain is reduced or eliminated.

Nursing interventions and rationales
1. Encourage the patient to increase her fluid intake.
Rationale: Additional fluids relieve pain by flushing the bladder.
2. Apply heat to the patient's lower abdomen or back.
Rationale: Heat promotes circulation, which assists in healing and encourages relaxation.
3. Administer mild analgesics, as ordered.
Rationale: Medications are sometimes necessary during the acute phase.

Nursing diagnosis
Altered Urinary Elimination related to infection
Desired outcome: Patient voids adequate amounts of clear yellow urine.

Nursing interventions and rationales
1. Monitor the patient's intake and output.

Rationale: Monitoring is necessary to assess urine output.
2. Assess the patient's urine for color, consistency, and odor.
Rationale: This assessment helps to evaluate the effectiveness of treatment and the amount of fluid intake.
3. Encourage the patient to consume sufficient fluids.
Rationale: Fluids dilute the urine and help to flush the kidneys.

Nursing diagnosis
High Risk for Injury related to the development of pyelonephritis
Desired outcome: Pyelonephritis does not occur.

Nursing interventions and rationales
1. Instruct the patient regarding the need for a full course of antibiotics.
Rationale: Antibiotics are necessary to eradicate bacteria.
2. Reculture the patient's urine after treatment; repeat at monthly intervals, as ordered.
Rationale: This procedure identifies failure of treatment and recurrence of infection.
3. Monitor the patient for signs and symptoms of recurrences of UTI and of pyelonephritis; instruct the patient in identifying these signs and symptoms.
Rationale: Prompt treatment minimizes complications.

Medical diagnosis
Medical diagnosis for UTI is based on urine culture (clean-catch midstream or catheterized specimen).

Medical treatment
Treatment for UTI includes:
• encouraging the patient to increase her consumption of fluids
• carrying out antibiotic therapy for 10 to 14 days. (*Escherichia coli* is the most common organism isolated; many strains have become resistant to penicillin. Nitrofurantoin has been advocated as a first-line therapy, provided the patient does not have glucose-6-phosphate dehydrogenase deficiency and is not close to term.)
• reculture after the treatment is completed
• monthly urine cultures obtained throughout the pregnancy (until delivery) to determine signs of recurrence.

3 Diagnostic Tests and Procedures

Here is an alphabetical listing of common diagnostic tests and procedures that you may perform or assist with during your clinical rotation.

☐ Alpha-fetoprotein (AFP)

Alpha-fetoprotein is a glycoprotein and a major component of fetal blood. With a highly vascularized, non-skin-covered defect (such as anencephaly and omphalocele), AFP concentrations in the amniotic fluid and maternal serum are greatly increased. The AFP test detects possible neural tube defects (NTDs) and abdominal wall defects. Recently, researchers have recognized the potential benefits the test has in identifying other perinatal problems (see below for specific disorders associated with high and low AFP levels). Two additional tests, unconjugated estriol and human chorionic gonadotropin (HCG), have been added to the maternal serum alpha-fetoprotein (MSAFP) test to improve the test's ability to identify the patient carrying a fetus with Down syndrome. This is referred to as MSAFP plus, triscreen, or triple screen. In Down syndrome, the MSAFP and the unconjugated estriol will be low and the HCG will be elevated. With the addition of these two tests, it is estimated that 60% of cases with Down syndrome can be identified. The best time to administer these screening tests is between 16 and 18 weeks; however, individual laboratories may extend this time frame to as early as 15 weeks and as late as 20 weeks.

Indications

• Many states now require that all women who enter the health care system early enough for screening have the opportunity to be tested.
• Diabetics have a higher incidence of such congenital defects as NTDs and should be screened. (Some research shows consistently lower MSAFP values in diabetic women.)
• Patients who have a family history of NTD or a child affected with the defect should be screened.

Contraindications

None

Interventions

1. Thoroughly explain the reason for the testing.
2. Obtain the patient's informed consent.

3. If amniocentesis will be performed, thoroughly explain the procedure and the risks to the patient (see "Amniocentesis").
4. After a specimen has been obtained, be sure to include the patient's race, weight, and history of maternal disorders (especially diabetes) as well as the gestational age of the fetus with the sample. These factors have been shown to influence MSAFP levels.
5. Observe the venipuncture site for bleeding.
6. Provide emotional support while awaiting results.
7. Provide appropriate counseling and referral for further testing for high and low values.

The following disorders may be associated with *elevated* MSAFP levels:

Maternal
• multiple gestation
• threatened abortion
• intrauterine fetal distress or death
• Rh disease
• ectopic pregnancy
• hepatitis
• hepatoma, GI cancer, and tumor metastatis to liver
• herpes infection
• pregnancy-induced hypertension

Fetal
• congenital cirrhosis
• NTDs
• sacrococcygeal teratoma
• omphalocele
• hepatitis
• fetal nephrosis and Potter's syndrome
• esophageal atresia
• growth retardation
• Turner's syndrome.

The following disorders may be associated with *low* MSAFP levels:
• Down syndrome
• insulin-dependent diabetes mellitus.

☐ Amniocentesis

The transabdominal removal of amniotic fluid from the uterus, amniocentesis is performed while the patient is under local anesthesthia, under the guidance of ultrasound to prevent injury to fetal or maternal tissues. The procedure is usually not performed before 14 weeks' gestation because of inadequate amniotic fluid volume.

Indications
• Prenatal diagnosis of congenital disorders
• Determination of the sex of the fetus in patients who are at risk for having children with sex-linked disorders (such as hemophilia)
• Determination of the bilirubin level of the amniotic fluid in Rh-sensitized pregnancies
• Estimation of fetal maturity
• Determination of the presence of infection
• Determination of the color of the amniotic fluid
• Relief of polyhydramnios
• Intrauterine transfusions and other fetal therapy
• Therapeutic abortion during the second trimester

Contraindications
• Anterior placenta with inadequate access to amniotic fluid
• Oligohydramnios

Interventions
1. Arrange for appropriate genetic counseling if amniocentesis is being performed to diagnose congenital disorders.
2. Explain the purpose and the technical aspects of the procedure to the patient.
3. Explain the risks of amniocentesis, including septic abortion, fetal or placental trauma, fetal skin scars, rupture of the membranes, pre-term labor, bleeding, and Rh-sensitization. The risk of pregnancy loss related to midtrimester amniocentesis is less than 1%.
4. Obtain the patient's informed consent.
5. Record vital signs, including fetal heart tones.
6. Note the patient's blood type and Rh factor.
7. Just before the procedure, have the patient empty her bladder.
8. Observe the patient for signs of supine vena cava syndrome, including nausea, dizziness, and diaphoresis.
9. During the procedure, assist as necessary and appropriate. The insertion site will be determined by ultrasound, and the skin prepared with antiseptic solution; a sterile field will be established.
   After a local anesthetic is injected into the skin, the needle is inserted into the amniotic cavity and the necessary amount of amniotic fluid is removed. Specimens are then labeled and transported to the laboratory.
10. After the procedure, the needle puncture site should be dressed with a small bandage, and the patient should remain under observation for at least 30 minutes.
11. To monitor for complications, check vital signs, including fetal heart tones, during the observation period.
12. Review with the client the signs and symptoms of complications, including bleeding, fluid leakage, pain, contractions, fever, and change in fetal activity; also review appropriate actions to take if complications occur.

13. Administer Rh immune globulin if the patient is Rh-negative.
14. Explain to the patient when the diagnostic studies will be completed and how she will be notified of the results.
15. Provide emotional support while the patient and her family are awaiting results.
16. Arrange for appropriate counseling and referral if the patient requires further testing or medical interventions.

☐ Amniotomy

Amniotomy, the artificial rupture of the amniotic membrane, is performed by inserting a device into the amniotic sac that tears the membrane, thereby allowing the amniotic fluid to escape.

Indications
• Induction of labor
• Detection of meconium-stained fluid
• Speeding of the labor process
• Application of a fetal scalp electrode
• Insertion of an internal pressure catheter to monitor uterine activity
• Obtaining fetal scalp blood

Contraindications
• High presenting part
• Unripe cervix

Interventions
1. Explain to the patient the nature and purpose of the procedure.
2. Place absorbent padding under the patient's hips.
3. Place the patient in the dorsal lithotomy position, with her knees flexed and body properly draped to avoid exposure.
4. Assist the health care provider during the vaginal examination.
5. After the procedure, immediately auscultate for fetal heart tones (or observe the monitor strip) and repeat the auscultation again in 5 minutes to rule out cord prolapse.
6. Note and record the exact time the membranes were ruptured. (Prolonged rupture of the membranes carries an increased risk of infection for both the mother and newborn.)
7. Note the color of the amniotic fluid:
• Meconium-stained fluid may be associated with fetal distress. The health care provider will need a DeLee mucus trap at delivery for suctioning. Specialized personnel should be present to suction meconium in the respiratory tract.
• Bloody fluid may indicate abruptio placentae or fetal trauma.
8. Note the amount of amniotic fluid:
• Polyhydramnios is associated with maternal diabetes and certain congenital disorders, especially those that prevent fetal swallowing (such as esophageal atresia).

• Oligohydramnios is associated with intrauterine growth retardation (IUGR), post-date pregnancies, and with certain congenital disorders, especially those which prevent fetal voiding into the amniotic fluid (such as renal agenesis).

9. Note the odor of the fluid. An unpleasant odor is associated with infection.

10. Expect more variable decelerations after rupture of the membranes as a result of cord compression during contractions. (Amniotic fluid serves as a cushion for the cord.)

11. Inform the patient that she may need to limit her activity as a result of membrane rupture or the placement of internal fetal monitoring equipment.

☐ Biophysical profile

A test for fetal well-being, the biophysical profile combines the nonstress test (NST) with other fetal parameters assessed by ultrasound. Fetal breathing movements, gross fetal body movements, fetal tone, reactive fetal heart rate, and qualitative estimate of amniotic fluid volume are evaluated by ultrasound and scored with the NST.

Indications

• A positive contraction stress test (CST) or a nonreactive NST may be an indication for a biophysical profile.

• Some institutions are using the biophysical profile in patients with premature rupture of the membranes (PROM) to identify subclinical chorioamnionitis.

• The biophysical profile may be used for primary fetal surveillance in high-risk pregnancies; however, the cost and the length of time required for the test make it impractical for routine use.

Contraindications

None

Interventions

1. See "Nonstress test" for specific interventions.

2. Note the following:

• Scores of 4 to 6 indicate that the test should be repeated in 24 hours

• Scores of 0 to 3 indicate the need for careful evaluation for delivery.

☐ Bishop score

Used to indicate maternal readiness for labor, the Bishop score is a method of evaluating cervical status and fetal position. Five factors are used in the method. These include cervical dilation, cervical effacement, cervical consistency, cervical position, and station of presenting part. Each factor is assigned a score of 0 to 3 and the total score is calculated; a score of six or more carries a 95% success rate for labor induction.

Indications
Before induction of labor for fetal or maternal indications

Contraindications
• Vaginal bleeding
• Ruptured membranes

Interventions
1. Explain to the patient the purpose of the procedure.
2. Place the patient in the dorsal lithotomy position, with her knees flexed and body properly draped to avoid exposure.
3. Assist with or perform the vaginal examination.
4. After the procedure, place a clean, dry pad under the patient.
5. Record the results.

☐ Blood glucose test (Dextrostix)
This test, which uses a heel stick, identifies hypoglycemia in the newborn. Hypoglycemia is defined as a blood glucose level less than 30 mg/dl (20 mg/dl for low-birth-weight newborns) during the first 72 hours of life, or less than 45 mg/dl after the first 3 days of life in all newborns.

Indications
Newborns at risk for hypoglycemia
• Birth weight greater than 8 lb, 13 oz (4 kg) or less than 5 lb, 10 oz (2.6 kg)
• Fetal asphyxia
• Intrauterine growth retardation (IUGR)
• Newborns of diabetic or preeclamptic mothers
• Newborns who are cold, septic, or polycythemic
• Severe erythroblastosis fetalis
• Congenital heart disease
• Newborns whose mothers received dextrose infusions before delivery
• Symptomatic newborns, such as those with feeding difficulty, apnea, irregular respiratory effort, cyanosis, weak, high-pitched cry, jitteriness, twitching, lethargy, or convulsions

Other newborns
• Many nurseries perform a blood glucose determination on all newborns during the transitional period after birth.

Contraindications
None

Interventions
1. Warm the newborn's foot to improve the surface blood flow.
2. Cleanse the heel with alcohol and allow it to dry.
3. Stick the heel in an appropriate site (see *Performing a heel-stick test,* page 51).
4. Remove the first drop of blood with a gauze square.
5. Position the foot in a dependent position to increase the blood flow.
6. After obtaining an adequate amount of blood, complete the blood glucose determination according to package directions. (Do not squeeze the heel too vigorously; it may alter test results.)
7. Cover the site with a small sterile bandage.
8. Record the results. A blood glucose level of 30 to 40 mg/dl is often treated with oral or gavage feedings to prevent further reduction in the blood glucose level. Newborns with profound hypoglycemia may require I.V. dextrose infusion. (*Note:* Heel-stick findings may be verified by blood glucose testing performed by a laboratory technician.)
9. Repeat the blood glucose determination after treatment for hypoglycemia.

☐ Chorionic villi sampling (CVS)
Chorionic villi sampling (CVS) is done during the first trimester, usually at about 8 to 10 weeks' gestation, to detect certain congenital disorders. Results are available within a few days (unlike amniocentesis, which may take 4 to 6 weeks for results).

CVS generally involves transcervical or transabdominal aspiration of fetal villous tissue. These tissues contain rapidly dividing cells that yield results much faster than the sloughing skin cells obtained during amniocentesis. Patients must be screened for vaginal, cervical, and pelvic infections before transcervical CVS to minimize the risk of infection.

Indications
Indications for CVS are essentially the same as for amniocentesis for prenatal diagnosis, except that CVS cannot be used to detect neural tube defects.

Contraindications
• Endocervicitis, genital herpes, pelvic inflammatory disease (PID), and positive cervical culture for gonorrhea
• Threatened abortion
• Cervical stenosis or incompetent cervix
• Maternal coagulopathy
• Rh sensitization

Interventions
1. Arrange for appropriate genetic counseling.

2. Explain to the patient the purpose and technical aspects of the procedure.

3. Explain the risks of CVS, including:

• spontaneous abortion
• infection
• bleeding
• premature labor
• amniotic fluid leakage
• premature rupture of the membranes
• contamination of the specimen by maternal cells.

4. Obtain the patient's informed consent.

5. Note the patient's blood type and Rh factor.

6. After the procedure, observe the patient for bleeding, leakage of amniotic fluid, and cramping.

7. Administer Rh immune globulin to Rh-negative unsensitized patients.

8. Instruct the patient to report bleeding, pain, leakage of fluid, myalgia, malaise, and fever (even low-grade fevers).

9. Provide the patient with emotional support while awaiting test results.

10. Arrange for appropriate counseling and referral if the patient requires further medical intervention.

☐ Circumcision

Circumcision is the surgical procedure in which the prepuce is separated from the glans penis and is excised.

Indications

Parental request

Contraindications

Circumcision should not be performed if the infant is premature or compromised, has a known bleeding problem, or is born with a genitourinary defect such as hypospadias or epispadias.

Interventions

1. Provide the parents with information regarding the pros and cons of circumcision.

2. Obtain informed consent.

3. Gather the equipment and prepare the newborn by removing the diaper and placing him on a circumcision board or other type of restraint. (Make every effort to minimize exposure of the infant because of cold stress.)

4. Provide comfort measures during the procedure, such as using a pacifier or stroking the baby's head. (Some health care providers use local anesthesia for the procedure.)

5. Following the procedure, hold and comfort the infant.

6. *After circumcision using the Yellen or Gomco clamp,* apply ointment, such as petroleum jelly, and gauze to the penis to keep it from adhering to the diaper. Repeat with each diaper change for 24 to 48 hours. *After circumcision using the plasti-bell,* keep the plastic rim in place for 3 to 4 days until healing takes place. (The bell prevents the penis from sticking to the diaper. The bell may be allowed to fall off or it may be removed by the clinician if it is still in place after 8 days.

7. Monitor the baby frequently after the procedure for bleeding. The infant should void within 4 to 6 hours of the procedure.

8. Prior to discharge, instruct the parents to squeeze water over the penis and to pat it dry after each diaper change. Observe the penis for bleeding and possible signs of infection.

9. Be aware that the glans penis becomes covered with a whitish-yellow exudate in 24 hours. This is part of the healing process and no attempt should be made to remove it.

☐ Contraction stress test

Used to indicate fetal well-being, the contraction stress test (CST), or oxytocin challenge test, involves external monitoring of the fetal heart rate and stimulation of uterine contractions by nipple stimulation or oxytocin infusion.

Although uterine contractions cause some hypoxic stress, a well-oxygenated fetus can tolerate such an insult, whereas a compromised fetus will demonstrate late decelerations. The presence of late decelerations may indicate placental insufficiency and fetal jeopardy; late decelerations appear to be an earlier warning sign of fetal deterioration than the loss of reactivity.

Negative contraction stress test

A negative CST is represented by no late decelerations of the fetal heart rate during 3 contractions in 10 minutes.

Fetal heart rate

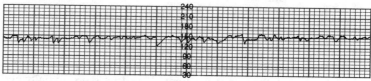

Contractions

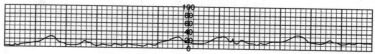

Positive contraction stress test

A positive CST is represented by late decelerations occurring in 50% or more of contractions in a 10-minute period.

Fetal heart rate

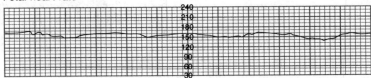

Contractions

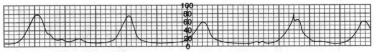

Indications

• Nonreactive or unsatisfactory nonstress test
• Some health care providers prefer to use the CST as the primary screening test for fetal well-being for post-date pregnancies, intrauterine growth retardation, and diabetes.

Contraindications

• Previous classical cesarean section
• Placenta previa
• Premature rupture of the membranes
• Twins
• Incompetent cervix
• Treatment of preterm labor
• Polyhydramnios

Interventions

1. Explain to the patient the procedure and the indications for testing.
2. Obtain the patient's informed consent as required by the institution.
3. Have the patient put on a hospital gown if I.V. oxytocin is to be used.
4. Place the patient in semi-Fowler's position with a slight left tilt to avoid vena cava compression.
5. Connect the patient to an external monitor.
6. Record the patient's blood pressure initially and every 15 minutes during the test.
7. Obtain a 10-minute strip to observe for spontaneous uterine activity.
8. Stimulate uterine activity with nipple stimulation or I.V. oxytocin (Pitocin).
• Nipple stimulation: The patient stimulates her nipples (according to individual hospital protocol) until a contraction occurs. In-

CONTRACTION STRESS TEST: RESULTS AND INTERPRETATIONS

Result	Interpretation
Negative No late decelerations of the fetal heart rate during three contractions in 10 minutes	A negative result is associated with fetal survival for 1 week. The test is usually repeated weekly but can be performed more frequently if indicated.
Positive Late decelerations occurring with 50% or more of the contractions in 10 minutes	A positive result may indicate fetal compromise. If the patient is at term, a trial of labor with optimum fetal heart rate monitoring is indicated. If the patient is not at term, additional testing may be indicated before the decision to deliver is made. (*Note:* This test carries a fairly high false-positive rate; a biophysical profile may be used in these situations.)
Suspicious Late decelerations with less than 50% of the contractions in 10 minutes	An equivocal or suspicious result indicates that the test should be repeated within 24 hours. If reactivity is absent, a biophysical profile is indicated.
Hyperstimulation Excessive uterine activity that causes late decelerations or bradycardia	If the result indicates hyperstimulation, allow the uterus to relax and restart the test at a lower dose or use less frequent nipple stimulation.
Unsatisfactory Inadequate uterine activity or fetal heart rate recording	If the results indicate an unsatisfactory response, the test should be repeated within 24 hours.

termittent nipple stimulation is continued until the patient has three contractions in a 10-minute period.
• I.V. oxytocin infusion: An I.V. is started and an oxytocin infusion is piggybacked into the primary line. The infusion is administered until the patient has three contractions in a 10-minute period.
9. Observe the patient closely for uterine hyperactivity; if uterine hyperactivity occurs, discontinue nipple stimulation or the I.V. oxytocin immediately.
10. To interpret results of the CST, see *Contraction stress test: Results and interpretations.*
11. After the procedure, observe the patient while checking the monitor until contractions subside.
12. Remove the monitor (and the I.V. if necessary) and inform the patient of the test results.
13. Schedule the patient's next CST or other procedures as indicated by the results.

☐ Deep tendon reflexes

Deep tendon reflexes (DTRs) are tested by striking a tendon (sensory impulse) and watching for contraction of the appropriate muscles. DTRs are increased in patients with central nervous system (CNS) irritability associated with pregnancy-induced hypertension. Brisk (3+ or 4+) DTRs suggest a worsening of the disease and the possibility of seizure activity. If the patient has a 3+ or 4+ DTRs, assess for clonus, which represents an increase in reflex excitability indicating severe CNS irritability. If the patient has clonus, she will exhibit rhythmic oscillations when the foot is dorsiflexed and similar oscillations when the foot drops to the plantar flexed position.

DTRs are assessed as follows:

4+	Hyperactive response
3+	Greater than normal
2+	Normal
1+	Low response, somewhat diminished
0	No response

Patients receiving magnesium sulfate therapy to decrease CNS irritability and to minimize the chance of seizures should have their DTRs checked hourly. If the DTRs increase or fail to return to normal (1+ or 2+), the patient may need more medication. Absence of DTRs in such patients suggests increasing serum magnesium sulfate levels that can cause cardiac and respiratory arrest.

Significant serum levels of magnesium sulfate (given in mEq/liter) are as follows:

4 to 7	Seizures prevented
10	Reflexes disappear
>10	Respiratory depression
12 to 15	Respiratory arrest
>15	Possible cardiac arrest

Indications

• Patients with pregnancy-induced hypertension
• Patients receiving magnesium sulfate therapy for pregnancy-induced hypertension or preterm labor

Contraindications

None

Interventions

1. Explain to the patient the purpose of the procedure and what she can expect.
2. Keep in mind that, if the patient has received a regional anesthetic, the biceps reflex may be used to assess DTRs.
3. Position the patient so that her legs are slightly flexed.
4. Support the leg under the knee; palpate the patellar tendon just below the patella.

5. Strike the tendon briskly with the pointed end of a reflex hammer.

6. Note the reflex extension of the lower leg.

7. Record the result on the chart.

8. Notify the health care provider if the DTRs are increasing or failing to return to normal levels during magnesium sulfate therapy.

9. Notify the health care provider if DTRs are diminished (1 +).

10. Discontinue the magnesium sulfate and notify the health care provider if DTRs are absent. Make sure calcium gluconate (20-ml vial of 10% calcium gluconate) is available if an antidote for magnesium sulfate overdose is needed.

☐ Diabetic screening test (glucose screen)

Used to screen patients for possible gestational diabetes (glucose intolerance during pregnancy), the diabetic screening test is a timed blood test to measure carbohydrate metabolism after a measured amount of glucose has been ingested.

Indications

The test is usually recommended for all pregnant patients between 24 and 28 weeks' gestation. If screening is not routine, patients at increased risk should be tested. (Some institutions screen these patients early in pregnancy; if the results are normal, the test is repeated at 24 to 28 weeks' gestation.)

Patients having any of the following characteristics should be tested:

• age 25 or older
• family history of diabetes
• obesity (weighing more than 200 lb [90.7 kg])
• previous stillbirth
• previous newborn weighing more than 8 lb, 13 oz (4 kg) or present fetus that is macrosomic on ultrasound
• previous newborn with hypoglycemia
• persistent glycosuria
• recurrent urinary tract infection
• recurrent candidal (*Monilia*) vaginitis
• polyhydramnios (present or previous)
• chronic hypertension
• poor reproductive history (more than three spontaneous abortions)
• previous newborn with multiple congenital anomalies
• history of gestational diabetes in previous pregnancies.

Contraindications

Known diabetic patients

Interventions

1. Instruct the patient on the purpose of the test and the procedure.

2. Tell the patient that the test does not require her to fast but that she should not eat, drink, or smoke between the time the carbohydrate is ingested and the blood sample is drawn (1 hour).

3. Administer 50 g of carbohydrate (either as a commercial oral glucose preparation or the equivalent in food ingested within 5 minutes).

4. Collect a venous blood sample 1 hour later and place it in a 7-ml gray-top tube.

5. Note that urine collection is unnecessary because glycosuria is common in pregnancy as a result of the lower renal threshold for glucose.

6. Schedule the patient for further testing, if needed. Patients with a plasma value of 135 mg/dl or greater should be scheduled for a 3-hour glucose tolerance test (GTT). (Some institutions use a higher value to avoid unnecessary 3-hour GTT; however, some gestational diabetics will go undetected if a higher cutoff for further testing is used.)

☐ Epidural block

Epidural block is a type of regional anesthesia used to produce relief from pain during labor or delivery. A local anesthetic is injected into the epidural space, which contains the nerve roots as they exit from the spinal cord. The nerve roots are exposed to the local anesthetic, which blocks out painful sensations.

Indications
• Relief of the discomfort of labor once contractions are well established (usually with the cervix dilated at 5 to 6 cm in a primigravida and 4 to 5 cm in a multigravida)
• Certain maternal cardiac diseases in which maternal expulsive efforts in the second stage of labor are contraindicated

Contraindications
• Severe hypertension (preeclampsia, eclampsia, and chronic hypertension)
• Maternal hemorrhage or hypovolemia
• Acute and severe fetal distress
• Infection near the injection site
• Neurologic disease
• Some forms of maternal heart disease that cannot tolerate hypotension
• Previous back injury
• Anticoagulation or inadequate clotting mechanisms
• Allergy to local anesthetic

Interventions
1. Explain to the patient the benefits and risks of the procedure, and have her sign a consent form. (This is usually done by the obstetrician or anesthesiologist.)

2. Explain the procedure to the patient.

3. Check for allergies to local anesthetics.

4. Check the I.V. for patency and the I.V. site for signs of infiltration.

5. Record the patient's vital signs and note the fetal monitoring strip to rule out fetal distress.

6. Preload the patient with I.V. fluids, as ordered by the obstetrician or anesthesiologist.

7. Position the patient on the left side with her shoulders aligned and knees slightly flexed.

8. Assist the doctor with the necessary equipment.

9. Provide the patient with reassurance and support.

10. Assist with the procedure, as necessary. After the skin has been prepared and a small amount of local anesthetic injected at the proposed injection site, a needle is introduced into the epidural space. A test dose of anesthetic is administered through either the needle or a plastic catheter threaded into the epidural space and left in place if the epidural is to be continuous.

11. Begin assessing maternal blood pressure, pulse rate, and respirations every 1 to 2 minutes when the test dose is administered.

12. If the test dose produces warmth and tingling in the lower extremities but no anesthesia, the needle or catheter is considered properly placed and the appropriate amount of anesthetic agent is administered.

13. If a catheter has been inserted, it should be closed off and taped in place, thereby allowing for subsequent injections of a local anesthetic.

14. After the procedure, continue to closely monitor the patient's blood pressure, pulse rate, respirations, and anesthetic level as well as the fetal monitor tracings. (Anesthetics inadvertently administered to C_5-C_6 [total spinal anesthesia] will compromise respirations.)

15. Keep ephedrine readily available in case the patient develops maternal hypotension; profound hypotension can result from sympathetic blockade.

16. Maintain the patient in the left lateral position (which prevents supine hypotension) or alternate sides (to produce a more even pain relief).

17. Monitor I.V. fluids to prevent hypotension and fluid overload. Patients receiving oxytocin for labor induction are especially susceptible to fluid overload.

18. Keep a tongue depressor on hand at the bedside in case the patient has an epidural-related seizure (caused by I.V. injection of the local anesthetic).

19. Epidural anesthesia may slow the progress of labor temporarily and lengthen the second stage of labor by reducing maternal expulsive efforts. Its use also increases the incidence of forceps delivery.

20. Monitor the patient's output carefully and check the patient's bladder frequently, as epidural anesthesia may make the patient unaware of the need to void.

21. To provide analgesia for extended periods of time (up to 24 hours) after cesarean section, the anesthesiologist can inject such medications as morphine into the epidural space prior to removal of the catheter. Monitor the patient closely for respiratory depression (fewer than 12 respirations/minute) and pruritis. Both side effects can be effectively treated with naloxone.

22. After the epidural catheter has been removed, continue to observe the patient for urine retention and monitor the catheter (or needle) insertion site for signs of infection.

23. Inadvertent puncture of the dura may cause leakage of cerebrospinal fluid with resulting spinal headache. Report complaints of headache to the anesthesiologist or obstetrician.

24. When sensations return to the extremities, assist the patient with ambulation, as necessary.

☐ External version

External version is the external manipulation of the fetus from an abnormal position (breech, oblique, or transverse lie) into a normal (cephalic) presentation.

Indications
• Abnormal presentation that persists after the 34th week
• Absence of contraindications to the procedure

Contraindications
• Engaged presenting part (breech)
• Previous cesarean section
• Obesity
• Oligohydramnios or ruptured membranes
• Placenta previa
• Multiple gestation

Interventions
1. Explain to the patient the purpose of the procedure and what she can expect.
2. Obtain the patient's informed consent.
3. Take the patient's vital signs.
4. Note the patient's Rh factor; if she is Rh-negative, check to see if Rh immune globulin was given at 28 weeks' gestation.
5. Perform a nonstress test to evaluate fetal well-being.
6. Start I.V. fluids and begin tocolytic therapy, as ordered; these measures relax the uterus and permit easier manipulation of the fetus.
7. Assist with the procedure, as necessary and appropriate. During the procedure, ultrasound is used to evaluate fetal position

and placental placement and to guide the direction of the fetus. The abdominal wall is manipulated to direct the fetus into a cephalic presentation, if possible. The patient's blood pressure is monitored to identify vena cava compression. Monitor the patient for unusual pain.

8. After the procedure, perform a nonstress test to evaluate fetal well-being.

9. Observe for uterine activity, bleeding, ruptured membranes, and decreased fetal activity.

10. With Rh-negative patients, perform a Kleihauer-Betke test, as ordered, to evaluate fetal-maternal bleeding. Patients who have not received a standard dose of Rh immune globulin at 28 weeks' gestation should be given the dose after external version. The Kleihauer-Betke test will identify patients who need additional Rh immune globulin.

11. Instruct the patient before discharge about signs and symptoms to report to the health care provider.

☐ Fern test

A microscopic slide test, the fern test is used to determine the presence of amniotic fluid leakage.

Indications
Patients with complaints of fluid leakage

Contraindications
None

Interventions
1. Determine how long fluid leakage has been occurring as well as the amount and color of the fluid.

2. Examine the patient's underclothes for signs of leakage.

3. Explain the procedure to the patient.

4. Place the patient in dorsal lithotomy position on a surface suitable for performing a speculum examination.

5. Perform a sterile speculum examination (not a digital examination) or assist the health care provider, using a sterile cotton-tipped applicator to obtain a specimen from the external os of the cervix and vaginal pool. (Ask the patient to cough; this often causes fluid to leak from the uterus if the membranes are ruptured.)

6. Spread the fluid on a clean, dry slide, and allow it to dry thoroughly.

7. Examine the fluid under the microscope. A fernlike pattern indicates the presence of amniotic fluid.

8. Inform the patient of the test results.

9. Keep in mind that the plan of care will be determined by the test results (see "Premature rupture of the membranes" in Section 2).

☐ Fetal monitoring

The electronic fetal monitor (EFM) provides a graphic display of the fetal heart rate and monitors uterine activity by a digital readout and tracing. This type of monitoring is used to detect fetal distress and also to measure the duration and strength of uterine contractions.

The EFM can be either external (noninvasive) or internal (invasive), which requires rupturing the membranes, attaching an electrode to the presenting part of the fetus, and in some cases introducing a pressure-sensitive catheter into the uterus.

Baseline fetal heart rate (FHR) is measured between contractions. A normal baseline reading is characterized by a fetal heart rate of 110 to 160 beats/minute.

Baseline changes

Deviations from the normal baseline FHR include tachycardia, bradycardia, and variability patterns as outlined below.

Fetal bradycardia

Fetal heart rate is < 120 beats/minute (see the sample tracing below). Causes of bradycardia may include late fetal hypoxia, use of beta-adrenergic blocking drugs, prolonged cord compression, or congenital heart block.

Fetal heart rate

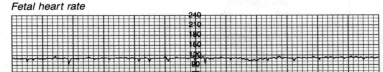

Contractions

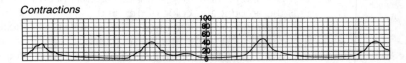

Fetal tachycardia

Fetal heart rate is > 160 beats/minute (see the sample tracing at the top of the next page). Causes may include early fetal hypoxia, maternal fever, use of parasympathetic drugs (such as atropine or hydroxyzine pamoate), use of beta-adrenergic blockers (such as ritodrine or terbutaline), chorioamnionitis, maternal hyperthyroidism, fetal anemia, or fetal cardiac arrhythmias.

Fetal heart rate

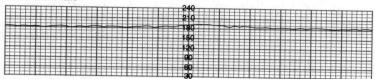

Contractions

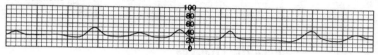

Variability
Variability refers to the change in the baseline fetal heart rate caused by interplay of the sympathetic and parasympathetic nervous systems. A fetal heart rate that fluctuates 6 to 25 beats/minute (average variability) at the baseline indicates a well-oxygenated, functioning central nervous system (CNS). (Internal fetal monitoring is necessary to evaluate variability accurately.)

Decreased variability
Fetal heart rate fluctuates 3 to 5 beats/minute (see the sample tracing at the top of the next page). Causes may include hypoxia or acidosis, use of CNS depressant drugs (such as narcotics or magnesium sulfate), prematurity, fetal sleep, congenital anomalies, or fetal cardiac arrhythmias. (Absent variability is 0 to 2 beats/minute.)

Fetal heart rate

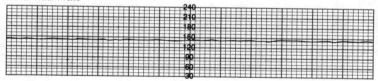

Sinusoidal pattern
Indicated by the presence of a uniform long-term variability with no short-term variability in the fetal heart rate (see the sample tracing at the top of the next page). Causes may include fetal anemia (Rh disease), severe fetal hypoxia before fetal death, or use of drugs (such as butorphanol tartrate).

Fetal heart rate

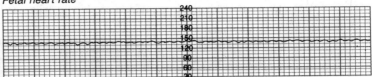

Contractions

Periodic changes

During fetal monitoring, *periodic changes* — accelerations or decelerations from the baseline — usually occur in relation to uterine contractions. Such changes are categorized as follows:

Early deceleration

Decrease in the fetal heart rate below the baseline; tracing shows a uniform shape and mirrors the image of the uterine contraction (see the sample tracing below). It is usually caused by head compression (vagal nerve stimulation); the fetal heart rate rarely falls below 110 beats/minute.

Fetal heart rate

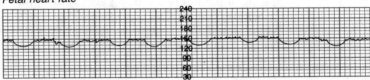

Contractions

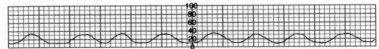

Variable deceleration

Abrupt decrease in the fetal heart rate, which is variable in duration, intensity, and timing (see the sample tracing at the top of page 179). Variable decelerations are usually caused by umbilical cord compression.

Fetal heart rate

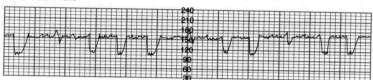

Contractions

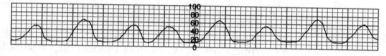

Late deceleration

Decrease in the fetal heart rate below the baseline; starts late in the contraction phase and recovers well after the end of the contraction (see the sample tracing below). This is usually caused by uteroplacental insufficiency.

Fetal heart rate

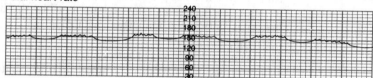

Contractions

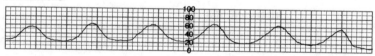

Uterine activity

When measuring uterine activity, the external monitor is useful for assessing the frequency and duration of contractions; however, it cannot be used to measure the strength of uterine contractions. With an internal pressure monitor the strength of uterine contractions can also be determined. The resting tone (between contractions) should be between 5 and 15 mm Hg; the time between contractions should be at least 30 seconds. The contractions should have an intensity of between 20 and 75 mm Hg and should last no longer than 90 seconds.

Hyperstimulation (characterized by inadequate relaxation, increased resting tone above 15 mm Hg, or peak contraction pressures above 80 mm Hg) may be caused by oxytocin administration, abruptio placentae, preeclampsia, or use of drugs.

Indications

External monitor
Routinely used for patients in labor

Internal monitor
• Decreased variability on external monitor
• Late or significant variable decelerations on external monitor
• Meconium-stained amniotic fluid
• Maternal complications that place the fetus at risk
• Dysfunctional labor, oxytocin induction, or stimulation of labor (indication for internal monitoring of uterine activity)
• Inability to monitor the fetus adequately with an external monitor (such as in situations involving maternal obesity, polyhydramnios, an active fetus, or multiple gestation)

Contraindications

External monitor
Patients in early labor and those experiencing a lack of progress in labor (such patients may be hampered by the limitation of maternal ambulation associated with EFM)

Internal monitor
• Active genital or cervical herpes
• High presenting part (a contraindication to rupturing of the membranes)

Interventions

1. Describe the procedure and answer any questions.
2. Obtain the patient's informed consent as required by institutional policy.
3. Take the following measures:

External monitoring (See *External fetal monitoring.*)
• Place the patient in semi-Fowler's position with the abdomen exposed.
• Cover the ultrasonic transducer crystal with an ultrasound transmission gel.
• Perform Leopold's maneuvers to determine on which side the fetal back is located and place the transducer over this area.
• Adjust the transducer until the best recording is obtained, and fasten the transducer with the elastic straps to the patient's abdomen.
• Place the pressure transducer over the fundus of the uterus and fasten it with elastic straps to the abdomen.
• Allow the patient to assume a comfortable position, avoiding vena cava compression.

EXTERNAL FETAL MONITORING

Tocotransducer
This features a pressure-sensitive button which, when placed on the uterine fundus, detects uterine activity. This activity is then relayed to the monitor, which records the frequency and duration of uterine contractions. The tocotransducer is usually used in combination with a fetal heart rate (FHR) monitor.

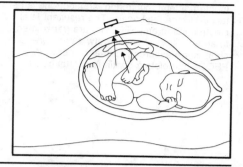

Ultrasonic transducer
This sends low-energy, high-frequency sound waves through the abdominal wall in the direction of the fetal heart. These sound waves strike the fetal heart wall and are deflected back through the abdominal wall (see arrows). The ultrasonic transducer then receives the deflected waves and relays them to the fetal monitor, which translates them into audible fetal heart tones and FHR waveforms. Because ultrasound reflects mechanical heart movement instead of actual electrical conduction, it is not as accurate as internal monitoring.

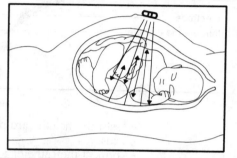

• Record the patient's name and the date and time on the monitor strip.
• Record on the monitor paper any maternal position changes, vital sign measurements, drug administration, and procedures performed.

Internal monitoring (See *Internal fetal monitoring,* page 182.)
• Place the patient in the dorsal lithotomy position and prepare the perineal area for a vaginal examination.
• Instruct the patient to breathe through her mouth and to relax her abdominal and perineal muscles.
• Assist the health care provider in placing the electrode on the presenting part.
• Apply a conduction medium to the leg plate and strap it to the patient's leg. Attach the electrode wires to the plate and plug the cable into the monitor.
• Label the fetal monitor strip with the patient's name and the date and time.

Internal monitoring of uterine activity
• Fill the uterine catheter with sterile water before insertion.

INTERNAL FETAL MONITORING

In internal fetal monitoring, an electrode is attached to the fetal scalp. The resultant fetal electrocardiograms (FECGs) are transmitted to an amplifier. Subsequently, a cardiotachometer measures the interval between FECGs and plots a continuous fetal heart rate (FHR) graph, which is displayed on a two-channel oscilloscope screen. Intrauterine catheters attached to a transducer in the leg plate measure the frequency and pressure of uterine contractions, which are plotted below the FHR graph.

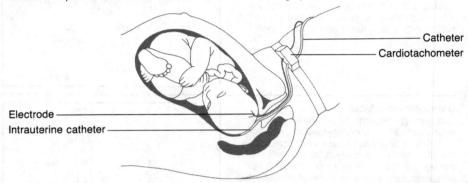

Catheter
Cardiotachometer
Electrode
Intrauterine catheter

- Assist the health care provider with placing the catheter in the uterus.
- Connect the catheter to the strain gauge, which converts the intrauterine pressure to an electrical signal.
- Tape the catheter to the patient's leg.
- Flush the catheter with sterile water every 2 hours during labor.

4. Record the baseline fetal heart rate, and take the following measures, depending on interpretation of the monitor test results:

Bradycardia
- Notify the health care provider if bradycardia occurs.
- No intervention is indicated if the fetal heart rate is more than 80 beats/minute and usually shows good variability.
- If decreased variability and late decelerations are noted, oxygen given at 10 to 12 liters/minute by tight face mask may be helpful.

Tachycardia
- Notify the health care provider if tachycardia occurs.
- No intervention is indicated if the variability of the fetal heart rate is good and usually there are no other periodic changes.
- If decreased variability and late decelerations are noted, take measures to reduce the patient's fever (if present) and administer oxygen at 10 to 12 liters/minute by tight face mask.

Decreased variability
- Notify the health care provider if decreased variability occurs.

• This is an indication for using an internal fetal monitor. (Variability cannot be assessed accurately with an external monitor. If variability is decreased on an external monitor, it usually is more severe than the tracing indicates.)

• If decreased variability is associated with fetal sleep or use of drugs, no intervention is required.

• Maintain the patient in the lateral position.

• Take appropriate measures to correct the patient's hypotension (if present).

• Discontinue oxytocin administration, if infusing.

• Increase the I.V. fluids.

• Administer oxygen at 10 to 12 liters/minute by tight face mask.

• Assist the health care provider with obtaining a fetal scalp pH, if ordered.

• Prepare the patient for operative delivery.

Sinusoidal pattern

If the sinusoidal pattern is a result of medications, no intervention is necessary. Otherwise, notify the health care provider because identification of the cause and appropriate treatment are essential to fetal well-being.

Periodic changes

• For variable decelerations:
  — Change the patient's position.
  — Perform a vaginal examination to rule out cord prolapse.
  — Discontinue oxytocin administration, if infusing.
  — Increase I.V. fluids.
  — Administer oxygen at 10 to 12 liters/minute by tight face mask.
  — Notify the health care provider if decelerations are severe and persistent.

• For late decelerations:
  — Notify the health care provider.
  — Keep the patient in the left lateral position.
  — Discontinue oxytocin administration, if infusing.
  — Increase the I.V. flow rate.
  — Take appropriate measures to correct the patient's hypotension (if present).
  — Administer oxygen at 10 to 12 liters/minute by tight face mask.
  — Assist the health care provider with fetal scalp sampling, if ordered.
  — Prepare the patient for delivery.

Hyperstimulation

• Discontinue oxytocin administration, if infusing.

• Increase the I.V. flow rate.

• Maintain the patient in the left lateral position.

• Administer oxygen at 10 to 12 liters/minute by tight face mask.

• Administer tocolytic drugs, as ordered, if the patient does not respond to the above measures.
5. After delivery, observe the neonate's scalp for signs of infection or abscess formation. (Some institutions apply antiseptic or antibiotic solution.)
6. Observe the patient during the postpartum period for signs of endometritis if an internal catheter was used to monitor uterine activity.

☐ Gavage feeding

Gavage feeding is the placement of a nasogastric tube in the stomach for the purpose of feeding the newborn.

Indications
• Premature infants, who frequently have poor sucking efforts (nipple feeding can cause tremendous energy expenditure)
• Hypoglycemic newborns, who may need rapid glucose administration
• Excessively tired or listless newborns or those who become cyanotic with feeding

Contraindications
Esophageal atresia

Interventions
1. Using a 15-inch #5 or #8 French feeding tube, measure the newborn for the distance to insert the tube. (Use the gastric tube to measure the distance from the newborn's ear lobe to the bridge of the nose to the tip of the xyphoid process.)
2. Restrain the newborn, as necessary.
3. To insert the tube, first flex the newborn's chin on his chest to facilitate passage of the tube by closing the epiglottis over the glottis. Then after lubricating the tube with sterile water, insert it through the mouth to the distance measured.
4. Check for placement by aspirating stomach contents or by instilling 0.5 cc of air into the tube and listening with a stethoscope over the epigastric region.
5. Monitor the newborn's heart rate and color.
6. After the tube has been properly placed, tape the tube to the newborn's upper lip, being careful not to occlude the nares. Then place the newborn on his right side with his head elevated to facilitate stomach emptying and to prevent regurgitation. Aspirate stomach contents to check for retained feedings if the newborn has been fed previously.
7. Allow a measured amount of fluid to flow into the tube by gravity (continuous drip via an infusion pump may be used). Then rinse the tube with a measured amount of sterile water.

8. During feedings, try giving the newborn a pacifier; nonnutritive sucking facilitates the body's response to the feeding and allows the newborn to practice the reflex.
9. Between feedings, remove the tube (as per institutional policy). Note that newborns who tolerate the procedure poorly may need to have the tube left in place. Keep the tube attached to the syringe barrel, leaving it open to act as a safety valve if vomiting should occur.
10. After the feeding, maintain the newborn in the same position for a period of time to facilitate retention and digestion of formula.
11. Monitor the newborn's heart rate and response to the procedure.
12. Recheck the newborn's blood glucose level if the procedure was ordered to treat hypoglycemia.

☐ Glucose tolerance test

A test that measures carbohydrate metabolism after ingestion of a measured amount of glucose, the glucose tolerance test (3-hour, 100-g carbohydrate) is used to confirm the diagnosis of gestational diabetes (glucose intolerance during pregnancy).

Indications
Patients with a plasma value of 135 mg/dl or more after a 1-hour 50-g carbohydrate screening test

Contraindications
• Known diabetic patients
• Patients with a 1-hour screening test with plasma levels approaching 200 mg/dl; values this high usually indicate glucose intolerance, and administration of a large volume of glucose may raise the blood glucose to dangerous levels.

Interventions
1. Explain to the patient the purpose of the test and the procedure.
2. Instruct the patient to ingest a diet containing at least 200 to 300 g of carbohydrate for 3 days before the test. (If carbohydrate intake is insufficient, falsely elevated values may occur.)
3. Instruct the patient to have nothing by mouth, except water, after midnight on the day of the test. Also instruct the patient not to smoke or exercise excessively for 8 hours before the test.
4. Obtain a fasting blood sample (use a gray-top tube).
5. Then have the patient ingest 100 g of carbohydrate (glucose) over a 5-minute period.
6. Obtain blood samples at 1, 2, and 3 hours. (Urine samples are unnecessary.)
7. Observe the patient for signs of hypoglycemia, including weakness, nervousness, hunger, and sweating.

GLUCOSE SCREENING FOR GESTATIONAL DIABETES

The following levels are considered abnormal for all pregnant patients regardless of age, weight, or duration of pregnancy.

Test	Serum (mg/dl)	Whole blood (mg/dl)
Fasting blood sugar (FBS)	>105	>90
1-hour	>190	>165
2-hour	>165	>145
3-hour	>145	>125

8. Encourage the patient to eat a balanced meal after the test is completed. (Instruct the patient to bring something to eat with her.)
9. Inform the patient of the test results, answering any questions and outlining a plan of care. If the fasting level is elevated or two other values are abnormal, the diagnosis of gestational diabetes is confirmed (see "Diabetes mellitus" in Section 2). For abnormal levels indicating gestational diabetes, see *Glucose screening for gestational diabetes*.
10. Patients with a normal 3-hour GTT should have a repeat 3-hour GTT in the third trimester.

☐ Induction of labor

Induction of labor is the nonspontaneous initiation of uterine activity to provoke the onset of uterine contractions that will result in progressive cervical effacement and dilatation with descent of the presenting part. Induction of labor is instituted when continuation of the pregnancy poses a serious threat to the mother or fetus or both.

Induction of labor may be accomplished by rupturing the membranes, stripping the membranes, inserting *Laminaria* into the cervix, using prostaglandin vaginal gel or suppositories, or administering oxytocin.

Indications
• Post-date pregnancy
• Any medical or obstetric complication that poses a threat to the mother or fetus, or both, if the pregnancy continues

Contraindications
• Fetal pulmonary immaturity (in severe complications the fetus may be delivered regardless of pulmonary maturity)

- Fetal distress
- Cephalopelvic disproportion
- Multiple gestation
- Placenta previa, abruptio placentae, or vasa praevia
- Uterine scar
- Abnormal fetal position or presentation
- Grand multiparity
- Macrosomia
- Bishop score of less than 6

Interventions

1. Explain to the patient the purpose of the procedure and what she can expect.
2. Obtain the patient's informed consent, if necessary.
3. For specific interventions associated with the procedure, see "Dystocia" in Section 2 and "Amniotomy" in Section 3.

☐ Kleihauer-Betke test

A quantitative assessment of fetal-maternal blood mixture, the Kleihauer-Betke test is used to detect the presence and amount of fetal blood in the maternal circulation.

Indications

Antepartum
- Hemorrhage (placenta previa or abruptio placentae)
- External version
- Symptoms suggestive of fetal-maternal transplacental hemorrhage

Postpartum
- Preeclampsia or eclampsia
- Cesarean section
- Manual removal of the placenta

Contraindications

None

Interventions

1. Explain to the patient the purpose of the test and what she can expect.
2. Obtain 3 ml of maternal blood in a purple-top tube. (Rh-negative patients who need Rh immune globulin will require one vial [300 μg] for every 15 ml of red blood cells [30 ml of whole blood].)

☐ Nitrazine test

The nitrazine test uses nitrazine test tape to detect the presence of amniotic fluid in vaginal secretions.

Indications

Patients who complain of fluid leakage

Contraindications

None

Interventions

1. Determine how long the fluid leakage has been occurring as well as the amount and color of the fluid.
2. Examine the patient's underclothes for signs of leakage.
3. Explain the procedure to the patient.
4. Place the patient in the dorsal lithotomy position if a sterile speculum examination is to be performed. (Do not perform a digital vaginal examination.)
5. Touch the test tape to the fluid in question. If the test tape turns blue-green, blue-gray, or deep blue, the membranes are probably ruptured. (*Note:* False readings can occur if blood, urine, or an antiseptic solution is present in the secretion.)
6. Inform the patient of the test results.
7. Keep in mind that the plan of care will be determined by the test results (see "Premature rupture of the membranes" in Section 2).

☐ Nonstress test

A noninvasive test used to determine fetal well-being, the non-stress test (NST) involves external monitoring of the fetal heart rate and observing the response of that heart rate to fetal movement. A fetus with adequate oxygenation, a functioning myocardium, and an intact central nervous system will accelerate its heart rate in response to fetal movement.

NST may be performed as early as 26 weeks' gestation; however, an extremely premature fetus may not give reliable results because of immaturity of the central nervous system.

Indications

• Previous stillbirth (testing should be started before the gestational age at which the last fetus died)
• Decreased fetal activity (or no fetal activity) noted for 8 hours
• Preeclampsia
• Chronic hypertension
• Intrauterine growth retardation

- Diabetes
- Post-date pregnancy
- Premature rupture of the membranes
- Abnormal fetal heart rate
- Sickle cell disease or other hemoglobinopathy
- Maternal heart disease
- Rh sensitization
- Renal disease
- Collagen vascular disease (such as lupus)
- Thyroid disorders
- All high-risk pregnancies

Contraindications
None

Interventions
1. Explain to the patient the procedure and the reason for the test.
2. Instruct the patient to eat before the test.
3. Obtain the patient's informed consent as required by the institution.
4. Place the patient in semi-Fowler's position with a slight left tilt to avoid vena cava compression.
5. Place an external monitor on the patient.
6. Record the patient's blood pressure initially and every 15 minutes during the test.
7. Interpret the test results based on the following:

Reactive nonstress test
Two fetal heart rate accelerations of at least 15 beats/minute above the baseline, lasting at least 15 seconds from the beginning of the acceleration to the end, in a 20-minute period (see the sample tracing below).

Fetal heart rate

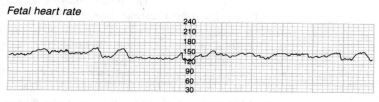

Contractions

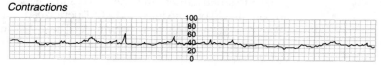

Nonreactive nonstress test

No accelerations or accelerations of less than 15 beats/minute or lasting less than 15 seconds (see the sample tracing below).

Fetal heart rate

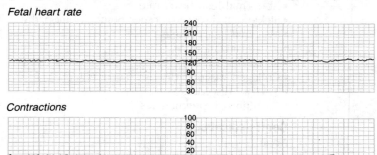

Contractions

Unsatisfactory nonstress test

No fetal activity or fewer than two movements in a 20-minute period.

8. Remove the monitor and inform the patient of the test results. Schedule the next NST or further testing as indicated by the results. Keep in mind the following information when scheduling the patient for subsequent tests:
• A reactive NST indicates that the fetus is likely to tolerate labor within 1 week. The test is usually repeated weekly; however, in certain situations, testing may be done two times per week.
• If results indicate a nonreactive NST, the patient should be scheduled for a contraction stress test (CST) or a biophysical profile the same day.
• Because the fetus may have sleep or inactive cycles lasting 20 to 40 minutes, a nonreactive test may be continued for an additional 20 to 40 minutes. The patient may be asked to eat a meal, then return for repeat testing. Alternatively, testing may include manual or acoustic stimulation (using an artificial larynx) to encourage fetal movement. If the fetus does not respond, the patient should have a CST or a biophysical profile the same day.
• Variable decelerations associated with fetal movement may indicate oligohydramnios, especially in relation to post-date pregnancies and growth-retarded fetuses. An ultrasound examination for amniotic fluid amount should be scheduled and a CST performed.
(Note: Some centers are incorporating fetal acoustic stimulation, using an artificial larynx to decrease the testing time and number of unsatisfactory tests.)
• Although many centers still have the patient indicate when the fetus moves, this is not necessary for test interpretation.

☐ Phototherapy

Phototherapy is the use of intense fluorescent lights to reduce serum bilirubin levels in the newborn.

Indications

Bilirubin levels greater than 10 to 12 mg/dl in a term infant or 15 mg/dl in a preterm infant

Contraindications

None

Interventions

1. Inform the parents of the reason for the therapy.
2. Obtain an informed parental consent according to institutional policy.
3. Expose as much of the newborn's skin as possible. (A surgical mask may be tied onto the infant as a diaper after removing the metal nose clamp if one is present.)
4. Cover the newborn's eyes with eye shields. Be sure the lids are closed when the patches are applied. Remove the shields at least once per shift to inspect the eyes for infection or irritation and to allow for eye contact with the parents.
5. Monitor the newborn's skin temperature closely.
6. Increase fluids to compensate for water loss.
7. Expect loose green stools and green urine.
8. Examine the genital area for skin irritation or breakdown.
9. Evaluate skin color with the light off every 4 to 8 hours.
10. Observe the skin for bronze baby syndrome, a grayish brown discoloration of the skin, urine, and serum in some newborns. Almost all infants recover from this with no complications.
11. Reposition frequently to expose all skin surfaces to light.
12. Provide tactile stimulation as often as possible. The newer phototherapy blankets permit parents to hold and feed their infants with the blanket in place.
13. Monitor serum bilirubin levels, as ordered. Progressive anemia can result from hemolysis of red blood cells.
14. After treatment, remove the newborn and continue monitoring for signs of hyperbilirubinemia. Rebound elevations of several milligrams are normal after therapy is discontinued.

☐ Scalp pH (fetal)

Assessment of fetal scalp pH involves obtaining a small volume of blood from the fetal scalp to determine a blood pH value.

Indications

• Significantly decreased or absent variability with no clear cause
• Persistently late decelerations with decreasing variability that have not responded to traditional treatment

• Unusual fetal heart rate patterns (sinusoidal pattern, tachycardia, or bradycardia) accompanied by decreased variability
• Maternal immune thrombocytopenic purpura (ITP) (performed to determine fetal platelet count and appropriate delivery route)

Contraindications

• Known or suspected blood dyscrasias (such as hemophilia)
• Early stages of a predicted long labor requiring frequent sampling because of an abnormal fetal heart rate pattern (Soft-tissue damage to the scalp may be considerable; cesarean section may be preferable.)
• Chorioamnionitis; a relative contraindication because of the possibility of increasing the risk of fetal scalp infection.
• Maternal HIV or hepatitis B infection

Interventions

1. Explain to the patient the procedure and reason for the test.
2. Obtain the patient's informed consent as required by institutional policy.
3. Place the patient in the dorsal lithotomy position with her feet or legs in stirrups.
4. Assist the health care provider with obtaining the blood sample. (The sample should be obtained before the next expected contraction.)
5. Prepare the blood sample to prevent exposure to atmospheric air, which could alter results.
6. Base interpretation of the test results on the following:

pH > 7.25	Normal
pH 7.2 to 7.25	Borderline; repeat sampling indicated
pH < 7.2	Fetal acidosis; delivery indicated

7. Assist with obtaining a simultaneous maternal blood sample, if ordered, to determine the patient's blood pH to rule out passive transmission of an abnormal state to the fetus through the placenta.
8. After the procedure, assist as needed and appropriate. The health care provider applies firm pressure to the puncture site through two contractions and continues to observe the site through the third contraction to assure hemostasis.
9. Reposition the patient for comfort and continue to observe for vaginal bleeding.
10. After delivery, inspect the infant's scalp to identify the puncture sites; continue to observe for bleeding and infection.
(Note: Recent research has supported the value of fetal scalp stimulation and fetal acoustic stimulation during labor to identify the truly asphyxiated fetus. These less invasive procedures rely on fetal heart rate accelerations in response to stimulation to identify the fetus who does not require scalp sampling.)

☐ Vaginal birth after cesarean section

Vaginal birth after cesarean section (VBAC) permits patients the opportunity of a trial of labor after previously delivering by cesarean section. In the past, health care providers followed the general principle that, once a patient had undergone a cesarean section, subsequent deliveries also had to be by cesarean section; health care providers feared uterine rupture of the old scar during labor. However, today, many health care providers are providing patients with the option of VBAC because of the serious, although rare, complications of operative delivery and the growing number of patients who want the opportunity to give birth without surgical intervention.

Indications
- Acceptance of the procedure by the patient
- Only one previous low-segment procedure
- Nonrecurring indication for a previous cesarean section (such as a prolapsed cord)
- Low transverse incision into the uterus
- Hospital properly equipped to perform a cesarean section in 30 minutes

Contraindications
- Nonacceptance by the patient
- Recurring indication for a previous cesarean section (such as severe cephalopelvic disproportion)
- Vertical, T-shaped uterine incision or lack of knowledge of previous incision type
- Any medical or obstetrical complication that increases risk for the mother or infant
- Macrosomia
- Previous uterine rupture

Interventions
1. Explain the advantages and potential complications of VBAC.
2. Instruct the patient to come to the hospital immediately when labor begins.
3. Have the patient sign an informed consent form according to institutional policy.
4. Assist with the procedure, as necessary and appropriate. The patient's blood should be cross-matched. A large-bore (18G) needle should be attached to the I.V. line to administer fluids rapidly, if necessary. Electronic fetal monitoring should be used. Uterine activity should be monitored closely using external or internal methods.
5. During the procedure, monitor the patient closely for unusual pain or abrupt changes in the fetal heart rate.
6. After the procedure, assist the doctor, as necessary and appropriate, to examine the uterine scar after vaginal delivery for evidence of separation.

Appendices

APPENDIX A: N.A.N.D.A. TAXONOMY OF NURSING DIAGNOSES

The currently accepted classification system for nursing diagnoses is that of the North American Nursing Diagnosis Association (NANDA), as shown in *NANDA Nursing Diagnoses: Definitions and Classification 1992-1993*. It is organized around nine human response patterns: exchanging, communicating, relating, valuing, choosing, moving, perceiving, knowing, and feeling. The complete taxonomic structure is listed here. The series of numbers before each diagnosis is its classification number, used to determine the placement of the diagnosis within the taxonomy. The number of digits delineates the level of abstraction of the nursing diagnosis (more specific diagnoses are assigned longer numbers).

Pattern 1. Exchanging (Mutual giving and receiving)

1.1.2.1	Altered nutrition: More than body requirements
1.1.2.2	Altered nutrition: Less than body requirements
1.1.2.3	Altered nutrition: Potential for more than body requirements
1.2.1.1	High risk for infection
1.2.2.1	High risk for altered body temperature
1.2.2.2	Hypothermia
1.2.2.3	Hyperthermia
1.2.2.4	Ineffective thermoregulation
1.2.3.1	Dysreflexia
1.3.1.1	Constipation
1.3.1.1.1	Perceived constipation
1.3.1.1.2	Colonic constipation
1.3.1.2	Diarrhea
1.3.1.3	Bowel incontinence
1.3.2	Altered urinary elimination
1.3.2.1.1	Stress incontinence
1.3.2.1.2	Reflex incontinence
1.3.2.1.3	Urge incontinence
1.3.2.1.4	Functional incontinence
1.3.2.1.5	Total incontinence
1.3.2.2	Urinary retention
1.4.1.1	Altered (specify type) tissue perfusion (renal, cerebral, cardiopulmonary, gastrointestinal, peripheral)
1.4.1.2.1	Fluid volume excess
1.4.1.2.2.1	Fluid volume deficit
1.4.1.2.2.2	High risk for fluid volume deficit
1.4.2.1	Decreased cardiac output
1.5.1.1	Impaired gas exchange
1.5.1.2	Ineffective airway clearance
1.5.1.3	Ineffective breathing pattern
1.5.1.3.1	Inability to sustain spontaneous ventilation
1.5.1.3.2	Dysfunctional ventilatory weaning response
1.6.1	High risk for injury
1.6.1.1	High risk for suffocation
1.6.1.2	High risk for poisoning
1.6.1.3	High risk for trauma

N.A.N.D.A. TAXONOMY OF NURSING DIAGNOSES *(continued)*

Pattern 1.   Exchanging (Mutual giving and receiving) *(continued)*
1.6.1.4   High risk for aspiration
1.6.1.5   High risk for disuse syndrome
1.6.2   Altered protection
1.6.2.1   Impaired tissue integrity
1.6.2.1.1   Altered oral mucous membrane
1.6.2.1.2.1   Impaired skin integrity
1.6.2.1.2.2   High risk for impaired skin integrity

Pattern 2.   Communicating (Sending messages)
2.1.1.1   Impaired verbal communication

Pattern 3.   Relating (Establishing bonds)
3.1.1   Impaired social interaction
3.1.2   Social isolation
3.2.1   Altered role performance
3.2.1.1.1   Altered parenting
3.2.1.1.2   High risk for altered parenting
3.2.1.2.1   Sexual dysfunction
3.2.2   Altered family processes
3.2.2.1   Caregiver role strain
3.2.2.2   High risk for caregiver role strain
3.2.3.1   Parental role conflict
3.3   Altered sexuality patterns

Pattern 4.   Valuing (Assigning relative worth)
4.1.1   Spiritual distress (distress of the human spirit)

Pattern 5.   Choosing (Selecting alternatives)
5.1.1.1   Ineffective individual coping
5.1.1.1.1   Impaired adjustment
5.1.1.1.2   Defensive coping
5.1.1.1.3   Ineffective denial
5.1.2.1.1   Ineffective family coping: Disabling
5.1.2.1.2   Ineffective family coping: Compromised
5.1.2.2   Family coping: Potential for growth
5.2.1   Ineffective management of therapeutic regimen (individual)
5.2.1.1   Noncompliance (specify)
5.3.1.1   Decisional conflict (specify)
5.4   Health-seeking behaviors (specify)

Pattern 6.   Moving (Involving activity)
6.1.1.1   Impaired physical mobility
6.1.1.1.1   High risk for peripheral neurovascular dysfunction
6.1.1.2   Activity intolerance
6.1.1.2.1   Fatigue
6.1.1.3   High risk for activity intolerance
6.2.1   Sleep pattern disturbance
6.3.1.1   Diversional activity deficit

N.A.N.D.A. TAXONOMY OF NURSING DIAGNOSES *(continued)*

Pattern 6.   Moving (Involving activity) *(continued)*
6.4.1.1   Impaired home maintenance management
6.4.2   Altered health maintenance
6.5.1   Feeding self-care deficit
6.5.1.1   Impaired swallowing
6.5.1.2   Ineffective breast-feeding
6.5.1.2.1   Interrupted breast-feeding
6.5.1.3   Effective breast-feeding
6.5.1.4   Ineffective infant feeding pattern
6.5.2   Bathing or hygiene self-care deficit
6.5.3   Dressing or grooming self-care deficit
6.5.4   Toileting self-care deficit
6.6   Altered growth and development
6.7   Relocation stress syndrome

Pattern 7.   Perceiving (Receiving information)
7.1.1   Body image disturbance
7.1.2   Self-esteem disturbance
7.1.2.1   Chronic low self-esteem
7.1.2.2   Situational low self-esteem
7.1.3   Personal identity disturbance
7.2   Sensory or perceptual alterations (specify visual, auditory, kinesthetic, gustatory, tactile, olfactory)
7.2.1.1   Unilateral neglect
7.3.1   Hopelessness
7.3.2   Powerlessness

Pattern 8.   Knowing (Associating meaning with information)
8.1.1   Knowledge deficit (specify)
8.3   Altered thought processes

Pattern 9.   Feeling (Being subjectively aware of information)
9.1.1   Pain
9.1.1.1   Chronic pain
9.2.1.1   Dysfunctional grieving
9.2.1.2   Anticipatory grieving
9.2.2   High risk for violence: Self-directed or directed at others
9.2.2.1   High risk for self-mutilation
9.2.3   Post-trauma response
9.2.3.1   Rape-trauma syndrome
9.2.3.1.1   Rape-trauma syndrome: Compound reaction
9.2.3.1.2   Rape-trauma syndrome: Silent reaction
9.3.1   Anxiety
9.3.2   Fear

APPENDIX B: UNIVERSAL PRECAUTIONS

When providing patient care, follow these Centers for Disease Control (CDC) guidelines:

Routine precautions

• Use appropriate barrier precautions to prevent skin and mucous membrane exposure whenever you anticipate contact with the blood or other body fluids of any patient. Wear gloves for touching blood and body fluids, mucous membranes, or nonintact skin of all patients; for handling items or surfaces soiled with blood or body fluids; and for performing venipunctures and other vascular access procedures. Change your gloves after contact with each patient.

• To prevent exposure of mucous membranes of the mouth, nose, and eyes, wear a mask and protective eyewear or a face shield during procedures that are likely to generate droplets of blood or other body fluids. Wear a gown or an apron during procedures that are likely to generate splashes of blood or other body fluids.

• Wash your hands and other skin surfaces immediately and thoroughly if they become contaminated with blood or other body fluids. Also wash your hands immediately after removing gloves.

• Take precautions to prevent injuries from needles, scalpels, and other sharp instruments or devices during procedures. Be careful when cleaning used instruments, disposing of used needles, and handling sharp instruments after procedures.

• To prevent needle-stick injuries, do not recap needles, bend or break them by hand, or remove them from disposable syringes. After use, place disposable syringes and needles, scalpel blades, and other sharp items in puncture-resistant containers for disposal. Keep such containers nearby. Place large-bore reuseable needles in a puncture-resistant container for transport to the reprocessing area.

• Although saliva has not been implicated in human immunodeficiency virus (HIV) transmission, keep mouthpieces, resuscitation bags, or other ventilation devices nearby to minimize the need for emergency mouth-to-mouth resuscitation.

• If you have exudative lesions or weeping dermatitis, do not provide direct patient care or handle patient care equipment until the condition resolves.

• If you are pregnant, strictly adhere to these guidelines. Although a pregnant health care worker is not at greater risk for contracting HIV infection than other health care workers, her infant is at risk from perinatal transmission.

Precautions for invasive procedures

According to the CDC, invasive procedures include the following:

• Surgical entry into tissues, cavities, or organs, and repair of major traumatic injuries in an operating or delivery room, emergency department, or outpatient setting (including a dentist's office)

• Cardiac catheterization and angiography

• Vaginal and cesarean delivery as well as other invasive obstetric procedures during which bleeding may occur

• Manipulation, cutting, or removal of oral or perioral tissues, including tooth structures, during which bleeding may occur.

For invasive procedures, follow these additional precautions:

• Use barrier precautions with all patients. Always wear gloves and a surgical mask. If blood or body fluids may splash or bone chips may fly, wear an apron or a gown and protective eyewear or a face shield.

• Wear gloves and a gown when handling the placenta or an infant during vaginal or cesarean delivery until blood and amniotic fluid have been removed from the infant's skin. Wear gloves while caring for the umbilical cord after delivery.

• If your glove tears or a needle sticks you, remove the old glove and put on a new one as quickly as possible. Remove the needle or instrument from the sterile field.

Source: U.S. Department of Health and Human Services. Centers for Disease Control. February 1989. *Guidelines for Prevention of Transmission of HIV and HBV to Health-Care and Public-Safety Workers* and U.S. Department of Labor. Occupational Safety and Health Administration, December 1991. *Occupational Exposure to Bloodborne Pathogens: Final Rule.* Washington, DC: Government Printing Office.

APPENDIX C: TIME MANAGEMENT SCHEDULE

	Monday	Tuesday	Wednesday	Thursday	Friday	Saturday	Sunday
6:00-7:00 A.M.							
7:00-8:00 A.M.							
8:00-9:00 A.M.							
9:00-10:00 A.M.							
10:00-11:00 A.M.							
11:00 A.M.-12:00 noon							
12:00 noon-1:00 P.M.							
1:00-2:00 P.M.							
2:00-3:00 P.M.							
3:00-4:00 P.M.							
4:00-5:00 P.M.							
5:00-6:00 P.M.							
6:00-7:00 P.M.							
7:00-8:00 P.M.							
8:00-9:00 P.M.							
9:00-10:00 P.M.							
10:00 P.M.-6:00 A.M.							

Source: *Guide to Surviving Nursing School.* Springhouse, Pa.: Springhouse Corp., 1991.

Selected References

Carpenito, L. *Nursing Diagnosis: Application to Clinical Practice,* 5th ed. Philadelphia: J.B. Lippincott Co., 1993.

Creasy, R., *Maternal-Fetal Medicine: Principles and Practice,* 3rd ed. Philadelphia: W.B. Saunders Co., 1994.

Cunningham, F.G., et. al. *Williams' Obstetrics,* 19th ed. East Norwalk, Conn.: Appleton-Lange, 1993.

Doenges, E.M., et al. *Nursing Care Plans: Guidelines for Planning and Documentation,* 3rd ed. Philadelphia: F.A. Davis Co., 1993.

Ferris, T. *Medical Complications During Pregnancy,* 3rd ed. Philadelphia: W.B. Saunders Co., 1988.

Freeman, R., Garite, T., et. al. *Fetal Heart Rate Monitoring,* 2nd ed. Baltimore: Williams & Wilkins Co., 1991.

Illustrated Guide to Diagnostic Tests. Springhouse, Pa.: Springhouse Corp., 1993.

Knuppel, R., and Drukker, J. *High-Risk Pregnancy: A Team Approach.* 2nd ed. Philadelphia: W.B. Saunders Co., 1993.

Nursing Student's Guide to Drugs. Springhouse, Pa.: Springhouse Corp., 1992.

Reeder, S.J., Martin, L.L., and Koniak, D. *Maternity Nursing: Family, Newborn, and Women's Health Care,* 17th ed. Philadelphia: J.B. Lippincott Co., 1992.

Springhouse Drug Reference. Springhouse, Pa.: Springhouse Corp., 1988.

Index

i refers to an illustration; t refers to a table

i refers to an illustration; t refers to a table

i refers to an illustration; t refers to a table